中 英 对 照
Chinese-English Edition

小针刀

陈小刚　主编
Chen Xiaogang　Chief Editor

治疗常见筋伤疾病

Acupotomy Therapy for Common Diseases of Soft Tissue Injury

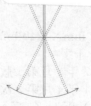

U0271314

广西科学技术出版社

图书在版编目（CIP）数据

小针刀治疗常见筋伤疾病：英汉对照 / 陈小刚主编. ——
南宁：广西科学技术出版社，2017.3（2024.4 重印）
ISBN 978 - 7 - 5551 - 0746 - 0

Ⅰ. ①小… Ⅱ. ①陈… Ⅲ. ①筋伤疾病—针刀疗法—
汉、英 Ⅳ. ①R245.31

中国版本图书馆CIP数据核字（2017）第 044417 号

小针刀治疗常见筋伤疾病
XIAOZHENDAO ZHILIAO CHANGJIAN JINSHANG JIBING

陈小刚　主编

策划编辑：罗煜涛　　　　　　　责任编辑：黄焕庭
责任校对：黎　桦　　　　　　　装帧设计：韦娇林
责任印制：韦文印

出　版　人：卢培钊
出版发行：广西科学技术出版社
社　　　址：广西南宁市东葛路 66 号　　邮政编码：530023
网　　　址：http://www.gxkjs.com

印　　　刷：北京兰星球彩色印刷有限公司

开　　　本：890 mm×1240 mm　1/32
字　　　数：110 千字　　　　　　印　　张：5.375
版　　　次：2017 年 3 月第 1 版
印　　　次：2024 年 4 月第 2 次印刷
书　　　号：ISBN 978 - 7 - 5551 - 0746 - 0
定　　　价：38.00 元

编委会成员简介
Introduction of editorial board

主编（**主译审**）：陈小刚，广西国际壮医医院、广西壮族自治区民族医药研究院、广西中医药大学附属国际壮医医院，骨伤科二级教授，广西名中医、医学硕士，2002 年赴美国学习，曾参与编写并翻译《中医骨伤科治疗手法图解：汉英对照》（2003 年由上海科学技术出版社出版）。

Chief Editor（**Chief Translator**）：Chen Xiaogang, national second grade professor of orthopedics, Guangxi famous TCM（Traditional Chinese Medicine）doctor, master of medicine, works in Guangxi International Hospital of Zhuang Ethnic Medicine, also known as Institute of Ethnic Medicine of Guangxi Zhuang Autonomous Region, and International Hospital of Zhuang Ethnic Medicine affiliated to Guangxi University of Chinese Medicine. He studied in the US in 2002 and acted as a joint editor and translator for the monograph *Illustrated Therapeutic Manipulations in TCM Orthopedics and Traumatology*（*Chinese-English Edition*）, which was published by Shanghai Scientific & Technical Publishers in 2003.

编者：

Editors：

韦礼贵，广西国际壮医医院中医副主任医师（骨伤科）

Wei Ligui, associate chief physician（TCM orthopedics & traumatology）of Guangxi International Hospital of Zhuang Ethnic Medicine

1

陈红，广西中医药研究院中医副主任医师（针灸）

Chen Hong, associate chief physician（Acupuncture）of Guangxi Institute of Chinese Medicine & Pharmaceutical Science

李凯风，广西国际壮医医院中医副主任医师，医学硕士（内科）

Li Kaifeng, master of medicine（TCM internal medicine）, associate chief physician of Guangxi International Hospital of Zhuang Ethnic Medicine

王玉雪，广西国际壮医医院医师，医学硕士（针灸推拿）

Wang Yuxue, master of medicine（Acupuncture & Massage）, physician of Guangxi International Hospital of Zhuang Ethnic Medicine

黄强，广西国际壮医医院医师（骨伤科）

Huang Qiang, physician（TCM orthopedics & traumatology）of Guangxi International Hospital of Zhuang Ethnic Medicine

吕春燕，广西中医药研究院中医主治医师（针灸推拿）

Lü Chunyan, attending physician（Acupuncture & Massage）of Guangxi Institute of Chinese Medicine & Pharmaceutical Science

何永园，广西国际壮医医院康复师

He Yongyuan, rehabilitation teacher of Guangxi International Hospital of Zhuang Ethnic Medicine

译审：

Translators：

陈昭，医学博士（留学比利时），供职于广东省中医药工程技术研究院

Chen Zhao, PhD.（studied in Belgium）, working at Guangdong Province Engineering Technology Research Institute of TCM

杰拉德·哈里斯博士，美国亚历桑那州，凤凰城印地安医疗中心

Dr. Gerald B. Harris, II L. L. C., Phoenix Indian Medical Center, AZ. USA.

陈靖红，广西中医药大学，英语副教授

Chen Jinghong, English associate professor, Guangxi University of Chinese Medicine

吕其玲，美国亚历桑那州，凤凰城印地安医疗中心针灸医师

Lü Qiling, O. M. D. L. Ac., AZ Acupuncture and Herbs L. L. C., Phoenix Indian Medical Center, AZ. USA.

周红海，广西中医药大学骨伤学院院长，医学博士（留学英国）

Zhou Honghai, PhD. (studied in the UK), director, College of TCM orthopedics and traumatology, Guangxi University of Chinese Medicine

主编简介
Brief Introduction of Chief Editor

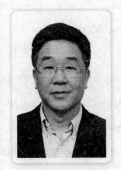

陈小刚，男，骨伤科国家二级教授，广西名中医，医学硕士。现任职于广西国际壮医医院（广西壮族自治区民族医药研究院、广西中医药大学附属国际壮医医院）。

1983 年毕业于广西中医学院。毕业后留校任教，并在附属医院骨科从事临床医、教、研工作。师从原广西中医学院院长、中国著名中医正骨手法名家韦贵康教授，曾担任其英语翻译。2000 年获骨伤专业医学硕士，2001 年 12 月获中医骨伤科教授职称。先后在广西中医学院（现广西中医药大学）及其第二附属医院、广西卫生管理干部学院和广西中医药研究院工作。2002 年曾赴美国辛辛那提大学学习，多次到美国、英国、德国、法国、捷克、泰国等国家和中国香港、澳门、台湾地区进行学术交流，曾被国家中医药管理局国际交流中心聘为"中医药国际交流专家"。

擅长手法、小针刀治疗骨伤科疾病，如颈椎病、肩周炎、腰椎间盘突出症、膝关节骨性关节炎等脊柱四肢疾病以及脊柱相关疾病；擅长用中西医结合方法诊治疑难性骨折、脱位、骨关节畸形、骨肿瘤等。

主持国家级和省部级科研课题 15 项，主编《常用中草药临床新用》，参与编写《中医骨伤科学》《骨伤科效方集》《中医骨伤科治疗手法图解：汉英对照》和《广西壮族自治区壮药质量标准》（第一卷、第二卷）等专著 10 多部，获得国家发明专利授权 6 项。任《中国中医骨伤科杂志》《中医正骨》《广西中医药》《广西中医药大学学报》等杂志编委，国家科技部中医药科技评审专家。

Chen Xiaogang, male, national second grade professor of orthopedics, Guangxi famous TCM doctor, master of medicine, works in Guangxi International Hospital of Zhuang Ethnic Medicine (also known as Institute of Ethnic Medicine of Guangxi Zhuang Autonomous Region, International Hospital of Zhuang Ethnic Medicine affiliated to Guangxi University of Chinese Medicine).

Graduated from Guangxi University of Chinese Medicine in 1983, professor Chen got teaching position in the same university, took responsibilities of teaching, medical work and research. He studied under professor Wei Guikang, a former president of Guangxi University of Chinese Medicine, and famous expert at manual manipulation of orthopedics and traumatology of TCM and was once professor Wei's English interpreter. Chen got his master degree of TCM orthopedics and traumatology in 2000, and obtained academic title of professor in TCM orthopedics and traumatology in December 2001. In that period, Chen worked in the second affiliated hospital of Guangxi University of Chinese medicine, then worked in Guangxi College of Cadre of Health Management and Guangxi Institute of Chinese Medicine and Pharmaceutical Science. Chen studied in University of Cincinnati of the US in 2002, and was invited by various institutions in US, UK, Germany, France, Czech Republic, Thailand, as well as Hong Kong, Macau and Taiwan of China for academic exchange. He was also appointed as international expert in Chinese medicine exchange by the international exchange center of State Administration of Traditional Chinese Medicine.

Professor Chen is specialized in therapis of manual manipulation and acupotomy for the treatment of spinal and extremities diseases in orthopedics and traumatology, such as cervical spondylosis, periarthritis of shoulder, prolapse of lumbar intervertebral disc, knee osteoarthritis and diseases related to spine; also good at diagnosis and treatment for complicated fractures, dislocation, deformity of bone and joint and bone tumour with combination therapy of traditional Chinese medicine and western medicine.

Professor Chen had taken charge of fifteen national or provincial research projects, published a monograph named *New Clinical Application of Common Herbal Medicine*, and acted as joint editor for more than ten monographs, such as *Orthopedics and Traumatology of Traditional Chinese Medicine*, *Efficacious prescriptions of Orthopedics and Traumatology of TCM*, *Illustrated Therapeutic Manipulations in TCM Orthopedics and Traumatology* (*Chinese-English Edition*) and *Guangxi Zhuang Ethnic Herbs Quality Standard* (*the first and the second volume*). He also gained authorization of six National invention patents and was appointed as member of editorial board of *Chinese Journal of Traditional Medical Traumatology & Orthopedics*, *The Journal of Traditional Chinese Orthopedics and Traumatology*, *Guangxi Journal of Traditional Chinese Medicine* and *Journal of Guangxi University of Chinese Medicine*, and evaluation expert at TCM science by National Ministry of science and technology as well.

前言
Preface

我们编写出版这本书，旨在帮助医师达到他们孜孜以求的目标：给予病人高质量的医疗服务。

小针刀诞生 40 年来，已经发展成为针刀医学，为众多的中医骨伤科筋伤疾病患者解除了病痛，从业者有十万之众，各类学习班星罗棋布，学员遍布中国各地，其中不乏外国学者。随着中医药对外交流的日益广泛和深入，针刀医学将进一步走向世界，我们特地编写了这本中英对照版的《小针刀治疗常见筋伤疾病》，向国内外读者介绍小针刀如何治疗常见筋伤疾病。

我们希望广大医师和医学翻译者，能感到此书对教学及临床确有裨益。如果大家认为《小针刀治疗常见筋伤疾病》对工作物有所值的话，我们呈献此书的目的也就达到了。

本书参考了国内的相关书籍以及英文医学书籍的翻译手法及风格，对前人所做的贡献，在此表示诚挚的敬意。

Our primary purpose in publishing this manual is to assist doctors in reaching the goal towards which they continuously strive: high quality medical service for patients.

Since its origin with over forty years of development, small needle scalpel therapy has become a branch of medicine, which known as Acupotomy and Acupotomology. It released patient's suffering from soft tissue injuries in TCM (Traditional Chinese Medicine) orthopedics and traumatology. More than One Hundred Thousand practitioners work in this area, and many varieties of training classes have spread across the country. Students came from many places including overseas. Acupotomy will reach further in the world with the spreading and deepening appreciation of TCM. This Chinese-English edition will introduce how the small needle scalpel therapy works for common diseases of soft tissue injury.

We hope that the many doctors and medical translators will find these pages a helpful adjunct to both classrooms and clinics. If professional doctors and translators find *Acupotomy Therapy for Common Diseases of Soft Tissue Injury* of value in their teaching programs, our objective in presenting this manual will have been achieved.

This manual refers to many works in the area, and also referred to the translation skill and style on English medical literatures. We wish to express our heartfelt thanks to those predecessors for their contribution.

目 录
Contents

◎第1部分　概论　Part 1　Introduction ·············· 1

1　小针刀疗法　Acupotomy Therapy（Small Needle Scalpel Therapy） ············· 2

2　针刀医学四大理论　The Four Great Basic Theories of Acupotomy ············· 3

3　治疗方法　Therapeutic Methods ············· 5

4　针刀四步操作规程　The Four Steps of Acupotomy Operation Instructions ············· 7

5　针刀针法　Manipulations of acupotomy ············· 10

◎第2部分　各论　Part 2　Monographs ············· 14

1　颈椎病　Cervical Spondylosis ············· 14

2　枕大神经卡压症　Greater Occipital Nerve Entrapment Syndrome ············· 25

3　肩胛提肌损伤　Injuries in Scapula Levator Muscle ········· 29

4 胸椎小关节紊乱症 Disorders of the Small Joint of Thoracic Vertebra ·············· 36

5 急性腰椎后关节滑膜嵌顿 Acute Lumbar Facet Joint Synovial ·············· 42

6 腰椎间盘突出症 Lumbar Disc Herniation ·········· 47

7 第三腰椎横突综合征 Syndrome of the Third Lumbar Transverse Process ·········· 54

8 腰椎椎管狭窄症 Stenosis of the Lumbar Spine ·········· 59

9 腰椎滑脱症与峡部裂 Spondylolisthesis and Spondylolysis ·············· 66

10 冈上肌肌腱炎 Tendinitis of Supraspinatus Muscle ······ 75

11 肩关节周围炎 Periarthritis of Shoulder ·············· 79

12 肱骨外上髁炎（网球肘） External Humeral Epicondylitis (Tennis Elbow) ·········· 86

13 桡骨茎突腱鞘炎 Tenosynovitis of Styloid Process of Radius ·········· 91

14 腕管综合征 Carpal Tunnel Syndrome ·············· 95

15 屈指肌腱腱鞘炎 Flexor Tenosynovitis (Trigger Finger)
··· 100

16 臀上皮神经卡压综合征 Superior Clunial Nerves
Entrapment Syndrome ······························· 105

17 梨状肌损伤综合征 Piriformis Injury Syndrome ········· 109

18 股骨头缺血性坏死 Ischemic Necrosis of the Femoral
Head ··· 113

19 膝关节侧副韧带损伤 Injury of Collateral Ligament of
Knee Joint ·· 120

20 膝关节骨性关节炎 Knee Osteoarthritis ················ 125

21 髌骨软化症 Chondromalacia Patellae ················ 133

22 踝关节陈旧性损伤 Obsolete Injury of Ankle Joint ··· 139

23 跟痛症 Heel Pain (Calcaneodynia) ················· 147

第 1 部分 概论

Part 1 Introduction

　　小针刀疗法是运用现代科学知识和方法，总结现代骨伤科关于软组织损伤和骨关节损伤方面的最新成就。在中医针刺疗法和外科手术疗法的基础上，小针刀疗法将西方逻辑思维运用于东方宏观辩证的哲学思想中，从而取得了突破性的成果。它是通过大量的临床实践总结出来的新疗法，既不同于中医针刺疗法，也不同于西医手术疗法，但它仍来源于针刺疗法和手术疗法，是针刺疗法和手术疗法的有机结合和发展。

　　Small Needle Scalpel Therapy, known as Acupotomy, summarizes the latest advancement in treatments of soft tissue, bone and joint injuries. On the basis of both TCM acupuncture and western surgery, Acupotomy Therapy combines the logical methodologies of western medicine with dialectical thoughts of TCM (Traditional Chinese Medicine). Through numerous clinical experiences, this new therapy not only shows its characteristics apart from acupuncture and surgery, but also represents an organic combination and development of its two origins.

　　小针刀是将针刺疗法的针和手术疗法的刀融为一体，把两种器械的治疗作用有机结合到一起，因此过去治疗学上一些难以解决的问题就解决了，一些难以达到的要求也达到了。由于新的思维体系出现，一些过去错误的病因病理观点得以纠正，含糊不清的病因病理得以明确和再发现，这使世界医学史又增添了新的篇章，诊断水平和治疗水平也上升到了一个新的高度。

　　Acupotomy merges needle of acupuncture and scalpel of surgery functions into a single whole. This integration solved some complicated problems that hinder therapy of related diseases. In addition, as the fulfillment of some previously difficult requirement, a new train of thought was generated, discriminations in cause and pathology corrected and confusions about some diseases were illuminated. Acupotomy opens a new chapter in the history of medical science, elevating diagnosis and therapy to a new height.

1 小针刀疗法 Acupotomy Therapy (Small Needle Scalpel Therapy)

小针刀疗法所解决的是一些常见病和多发病的诊断和治疗方法的问题，其中包括各种软组织损伤后遗症、部分骨刺、四肢陈旧性骨折后遗症、某些运动系统疾病所引起的后遗症，这些疾病严重影响了运动功能，使患者不能参加社会生产，从而加重了社会的负担。

The aim and utility of Acupotomy mainly focused on the diagnosis and treatment of commonly occurring diseases, including soft tissue injury sequelae, partial spurs, old fracture sequelae of limbs and sequelae of locomotor diseases. Such diseases severely affect motor function, making patients experience severe inconvenience in their daily work.

小针刀疗法具有方法简便、痛苦小、见效快、花钱少、变不治为可治、变复杂为简单、变难治为速愈等特点。

So, the acupotomy has many advantages, such as easy performance, less pain, instant effects and lower cost, which turned the incurable to curable, the complicated to simple and the difficult to quick healed.

小针刀疗法操作的特点：在治疗部位刺入深部到病变处进行轻松的切割、剥离等不同的刺激、松解，以达到止痛祛病的目的。

Features of Acupotomy: An acupotomy was inserted deep into the treatment site, which was then followed with a slight cutting and detaching of lesion tissue, which finally led to the relief and removal of pain and diseases.

2 针刀医学四大理论 The Four Great Basic Theories of Acupotomy

小针刀疗法的有关理论，是将中医针刺理论与外科手术理论进行融会贯通的结果。在此基础上，小针刀疗法的有关理论体系应运而生，形成了一个新的理论系统。这一理论系统以"四大理论"（闭合性手术疗法理论、慢性软组织损伤病因病理新理论、骨质增生新的病因学理论、经络实质新理论）为基础。在"四大理论"的指导下，针刀医学形成一个独具特色的治疗学体系。

The theory of Acupotomy is an achievement combining TCM acupuncture and surgery. Based on which, Acupotomy develops an innovative theory system, which can be categorized into four theories, namely, theory of closed surgery, new theories in etiology and pathology of chronic soft tissue injuries, new etiological theory of hyperosteogeny and new theory of the nature of Meridian. Such achievements can be used to guide acupotomy and form a unique treatment system.

（1）闭合性手术疗法理论：随着社会的发展、人类思想的进步，人类对疾病治疗标准的不断提高，要求既要解除致病因素，又要手术没有痛苦，不切开皮肤，没有损伤，不留后遗症，甚至要求不留疤痕。小针刀疗法正是在这一环境下应运而生的。它是一种闭合性手术疗法，是切开手术疗法过渡到闭合性手术疗法迈出的第一步。

Theory of closed surgery: Requirement of treatment is continuous and is developing along with the progress of society and philosophy that illness should be rooted without pain, cutting in the skin, additional injuries or sequelae and even without a scratch. The development of Acupotomology suited just such an atmosphere; it provides initial steps from excessive cutting toward closed surgery.

（2）慢性软组织损伤病因病理新理论：慢性软组织损伤的根本病理机制是动态平衡失调，其内涵主要是指它对人体内部运动器官的病理机制的概括和描述。

New theories in etiology and pathology of chronic soft tissue injuries: The disorder of dynamic balance is the fundamental pathological mechanism for chronic soft tissue injuries, which includes summary and description of pathological mechanism of motion organs inside human body.

（3）骨质增生新的病因学理论：骨质增生的根本原因是力平衡失调。根据这一理论，可将骨质增生分为压应力过高引起的骨质增生、拉应力过高引起的骨质增生、张应力过高引起的骨质增生三类。

New etiological theory of hyperosteogeny: Disorder of human internal force balance is the real reason for hyperosteogeny. Based on this theory, hyperosteogeny can be divided into three categories: hyperosteogeny caused by high compressive stress, by high pulling stress and by high tensile stress.

（4）经络实质新理论：针刀医学在临床实践中发现人体内存在着一个庞大的生理线路系统，其主要干线就是中国古代医学所描述的经络，即神经调节系统、生物电调节系统、体液调节系统和综合调节系统组成的人体信息反应系统。

New theory of the nature of Meridian: Acupotomology experience revealed the existence of a complicated physiological circulation in the body that the meridian acts as the main stream as TCM classics described.

Such anthropometric responses were comprised by regulation systems in nerves, bioelectricity, body fluid and integrated control.

针刀医学临床研究，支持了人体内经络系统的客观存在，主要线路的循行与中医经络系统的描述极为一致。

Acupotomology clinical research evidence supports existence of the meridian system of TCM theory inside the human body. The main lines are exactly the same as described in traditional Chinese medicine as the Meridian system.

（由美国亚历桑那州凤凰城印地安医疗中心的杰拉德·哈理斯博士审校）

（Revised & proofed by Dr. Gerald B. Harris, II L. L. C., Phoenix Indian Medical Center, AZ., USA）

3 治疗方法 Therapeutic Methods

小针刀是一种带刃的针，由针刃、针体和针柄组成。1976 年由针刀医学大师朱汉章先生在中国江苏省发明。

An acupotomy is a needle with a blade, which consists of blade, body and handle. It was invented by a great master of Acupotomology Medicine, Mr. Zhu Hanzhang, in Jiangsu province of China in 1976.

经过 40 多年的发展，小针刀疗法已经成为中医学的一个分支——针刀医学，涵盖经络穴位、神经解剖、生理病理、诊断与鉴别诊断、治疗技法与器械规范等一系列学科要素，并经过大量临床实践验证，成为一门具有现代中医特色的优势学科。

In its fortieth anniversary, Acupotomy has merged with TCM to become an indispensable branch. It has covered a series of scientific essence including meridian and acupoints, nerve dissection, physiology and pathology, diagnosis and identification, also treatment and instrument. Through large amount of clinical experiences, Acupotomy was proven to be a modern discipline with TCM features and advantages.

针刀有三种治疗作用：一是针灸针的刺激作用；二是刀的切割作用；三是针与刀的综合作用。针刀疗法是一种源于中医针灸的疗法，在针刺的基础上，对病变部位闭合性松解，通过解除筋经的粘连、痉挛或瘢痕，恢复机体的力学平衡，从而治疗脊柱和四肢筋伤疾病，以及脊柱相关疾病。针刀疗法具有方便、快捷、安全、有效、价廉等优势，尤其对颈椎病、肩周炎、腰椎间盘突出症等筋伤疾病具有显著的临床疗效，深受医学界和患者的欢迎。

There are three therapeutic effect of acupotomy: the effect of the acupuncture needle stimulation, the effect of the scalpel's cutting and their integrated effect. Originated from acupuncture, acupotomy can cut and detach adhesion, spasm and cicatrix of the abnormal tendon and tissues remove clog and restore dynamic balance of the body, thereby treating spine and limb muscle injury diseases and spinal related diseases as well. Acupotomy is convenient, safe, effective and economic, especially for patients with soft tissue injuries including cervical spondylosis, periarthritis of shoulder and prolapse of lumbar intervertebral disc. It received affirmative responses and acceptance from both medical professionals and patients.

根据不同治疗的需要，针刀有多种类型，但最常用的是平刃针刀，该型针刀有Ⅰ型、Ⅱ型、Ⅲ型三种基本型号，Ⅰ型又分为长短不同的四种，分别记作Ⅰ-1、Ⅰ-2、Ⅰ-3、Ⅰ-4（图1-1）。

To meet different therapeutic needs, numerous varieties of acupotomy can be applied. The most commonly used kind is the flat-blade acupotomy. It has three basic types: type-Ⅰ, type-Ⅱ and type-Ⅲ. As for type-Ⅰ, it has four models based on different lengths. They are named Ⅰ-1, Ⅰ-2, Ⅰ-3 and Ⅰ-4 (Figure 1-1).

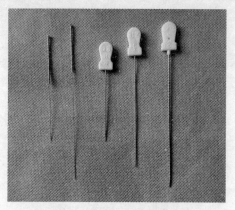

图 1-1 小针刀与针灸针

Figure 1-1 Acupotomy & Acupuncture needle

针刀分为柄、身和刃。柄为扁平葫芦状，厚度为 2 mm；针身为圆柱形，直径为 1 mm；刃为楔形，末端平齐，刀口线宽 0.8 mm，厚 0.2 mm。

An acupotomy consists of handle, body and blade. The handle is about 2 mm thick, flat, just like a calabash. The body is cylindrical shape with 1 mm diameter. The blade is subuliform with a flat tip. The tip is 0.8 mm wide and 0.2 mm thick.

4 针刀四步操作规程 The Four Steps of Acupotomy Operation Instructions

针刀的四步操作为定点、定向、加压分离、刺入。

They are location, direction, pressing to separate and insertion.

（1）定点：根据诊断制订治疗方案，选择进针点并用记号笔标示（图 1-2）。

Location: Create a treatment plan based on diagnosis, and then mark the inserting points (Figure 1-2).

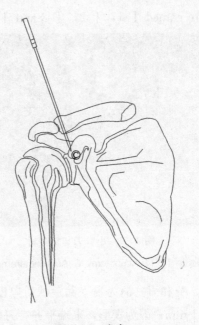

图 1 - 2 定点

Figure 1 - 2 Location

（2）定向：以针刀方向作为刀口线，一般进针时针刃方向即刀口线与进针部位的肌纤维、韧带、神经、血管循行方向一致（图 1 - 3）。

Direction: Inserted alongside the direction of needle's blade line which is usually parallel to distributed direction of the muscle fibers, ligaments, nerves and blood vessels under operating area (Figure 1 - 3).

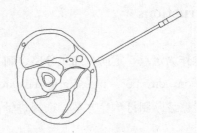

图 1 - 3 定向

Figure 1 - 3 Direction

（3）加压分离：为避开神经、血管，进针时以一手拇指或食指下压皮肤使之凹陷，针刀再沿指甲背进针。如有骨突部位，左手指压在骨突上，压陷皮肤及皮下组织后再进针（图 1-4）。

Pressing to separate：Avoid injuring nerves and blood vessels by pressing down the skin and separating tissue underneath with one thumb or index finger when needle is inserted. The operator keeps the needle tip close against his nail，and then inserts the needle into the point. If apophysis exists，the operator presses down the patient's skin and subcutaneous tissue with one finger，and then inserts the needle as mentioned above （Figure 1-4）.

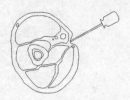

图 1-4　加压分离

Figure 1-4　Pressing to separate

（4）刺入：将针刀紧贴压在进针点手指指甲缘，快速穿透皮肤（图 1-5）。

Insertion：An acupotomy is inserted through the skin along while pressing the fingernail downward rapidly （Figure 1-5）.

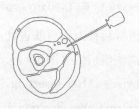

图 1-5　刺入

Figure 1-5　Insertion

5 针刀针法 Manipulations of acupotomy

（1）纵行疏通：进针后针刀以皮肤进针点为中心，针柄沿刀口线方向摆动，以疏通软组织粘连（图 1 - 6）。

Dredging lengthwise: After insertion, swing the needle at its back end around the insertion point, lengthwise along the edge line to release adhesion of the soft tissue (Figure 1 - 6).

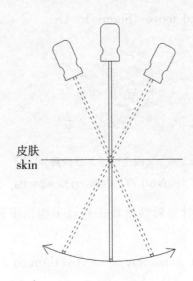

皮肤
skin

图 1 - 6 纵行疏通

Figure 1 - 6 Dredging lengthwise

（2）横行分离：进针后针刀以皮肤进针点为中心，针柄在刀口线垂直方向摆动，以分离瘢痕组织（图 1 - 7）。

Seperating broadwise: After inserting, swing the needle as part (1) described, except that the direction is perpendicular, which is used to detach the cicatrix tissue (Figure 1 - 7).

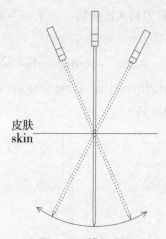

图 1-7 横行分离

Figure 1-7 Seperating broadwise

（3）多向透刺：进针某点后不用出针，针刀尖提至皮下，转向四周邻近组织或穴位透刺，以扩大治疗范围而不重复进针（图 1-8）。

Multidirectional penetrating：Inserting the acupotomy to subcutaneous level while turning the needle to surrounding tissue or penetrating accupoints for amplification of the treatment area without repetitively inserting through skin（Figure 1-8）.

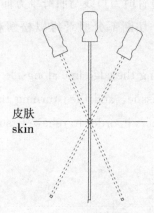

图 1-8 多向透刺

Figure 1-8 Multidirectional penetrating

（4）提插法：小针刀刺入皮肤后，一上一下地纵向进退的操作方法（图 1－9）。

Lifting-thrusting：After entering the skin，acupotomy is inserted down and withdrowed up along longitudinal axis of the body or the limb（Figure 1－9）.

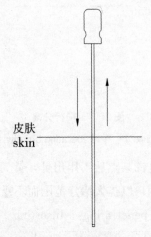

图 1－9　提插法
Figure 1－9　Lifting-thrusting

（5）横行切断：进针时刀口线与肌纤维方向一致，到达病变组织时将针刀口旋转 90°，切断部分肌纤维以松解粘连、解除痉挛（图 1－10）。

Cross-cut：Pointing the edge line alongside the muscle fiber until it reaches the lesion tissue，and then turning the edge line vertically to cut a few muscle fibers in order to relieve tissue adhesion and spasm（Figure 1－10）.

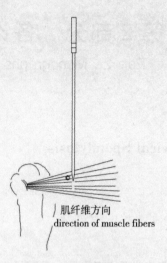

图 1－10 横行切断

Figure 1－10 Cross-cut

（由陈靖红审校）

（Revised & proofed by Chen Jinghong）

第 2 部分　各论
Part 2　Monographs

1　颈椎病　Cervical Spondylosis

【概述】Overview

颈椎病亦称"颈椎综合征"，是一种颈椎退行性病变，与颈部软组织慢性劳损、椎间盘退化有关，继而刺激神经血管等组织而出现颈肩臂痛、眩晕、手指麻木或运动障碍等一系列症状，是 40 岁以上人群的常见病、多发病。

Cervical spondylosis，also called cervical syndrome，is defined as a generalized disease affecting the entire cervical spine，related to chronic strain of cervical soft tissue and chronic disk degeneration，followed by stimulation of the nerve，blood vessel and other tissues，which brings about a series of symptoms，such as painful neck radiating into the interscapular area and into the arm，dizziness，numb or dyskinesia of fingers. It is a commonly and frequently encountered disease in people over 40 years old.

颈椎病的发生取决于脊髓与椎弓的关系，颈部的骨化病变实际上是继发于椎间盘退变的后纵韧带增厚并突出至椎管中，而椎间盘退变和骨性关节炎导致脊髓和神经根损伤。

The occurrence of cervical spondylosis relates to the relationship between the spinal cord and its bony arcade which has been studied extensively. Spondylotic lesion in cervical region is actually a thickened posterior longitudinal ligament protruding into the canal secondary to disk degeneration. Disk degeneration and osteoarthritis could lead to cord and nerve root impingement.

脊髓前动脉因椎间盘而受损也是病变之一。椎间盘退变始于纤维环后外侧撕裂，髓核水分和蛋白多糖的丢失使间盘高度减少。纵向韧带退变和形成的骨赘侵入椎体，形成硬化的椎间盘从而影响到椎管和椎间孔。最易受影响的节段是活动较多的第五至第六颈椎（C5～C6）、第四至第七颈椎（C4～C7）和第四至第五颈椎（C4～C5）。颈椎间盘间隙收缩可以因为黄韧带的变形，进而使椎管更加狭窄。节段性不稳将引起钩椎关节和小关节骨赘形成，这些突出物将同时压迫椎间孔和椎管。

Concurrently, anterior spinal artery impingement by the disk was proposed as part of the phthogenesis. Disk degeneration starts with tears in the posterolateral region of the annulus. The subsequent loss of water content and proteoglycans in the nucleus then leads to a decrease of disk height. The longitudinal ligaments degenerate and form bony spurs at their insertion into the vertebral body. These so-called hard disks have to be distinguished from soft disks, which represent acute herniation of disk material into the spinal canal or into the neural foramen. The most frequently involved levels are the more mobile segments C5～C6, C4～C7 and C4～C5. The converging of the cervical disk space may result in buckling of the ligamentum flavum, with further narrowing of the spinal canal. Segmental instability will result in hypertrophic formation of osteophytes by the uncoertebral joint of Luschka and by the facet joints. These prominent spurs will compress both the neural foramina and the spinal canal.

脊髓型颈椎病的颈椎椎管矢状径明显比正常者小（平均小

15

3 mm)。通过对比发现发病前后颈椎椎管形状有变化，颈椎在后伸位椎间孔明显变小。

The measurement of the sagittal cervical canal diameter was appreciably smaller (as much as 3 mm) in the myelopathic Spondylitic spine when compared to normal healthy spines. Comparing cervical canal size with onset of myelopathy in the cervical spine undergoing spondylitic changes，there is marked narrowing of the neuroforamen significantly in the extension position of the cervical spine.

【诊断要点】Keys to Diagnosis

（1）颈痛或伴头痛、肩背痛、臂（上臂或前臂）或手某部位的定位性疼痛或麻木，脸、颈、肩、上肢的某块或某局部肌肉跳动（痉挛）。

Signs and symptoms include neck pain with the association of the following symptoms：headache，pain in shoulders，back pain，pain in bilateral upper extremities (including arms and forearms). Or the pain can be localized to particular region of the hand. This pain can also include numbness. Complaint also includes the spasms of muscles in the face or neck，shoulders or either upper extremity's.

（2）头晕或眩晕、视力障碍或易疲劳，耳鸣失听，心悸（心率过快或过慢），血压改变（高血压或低血压），多汗或无汗，咽部有异物感，鼻塞和流涕交替出现。

Clinical findings may include：Dizziness or vertigo，vision disorder or eye tiredness，tinnitus and hearing loss，palpitate (tachycardia or bradycadia)，dysarteriotony (hypertension or hypotension)，hidrosis or adhidrosis，foreign body sensation in pharynx，stuffy nose and running nose alternately.

（3）下肢发僵、无力，行走时有似踩棉花感；某一肢体，或双上

16

肢，或双下肢，或交叉上下肢，或四肢出现不同程度的瘫痪。

Muscle rigidity and weakness of the lower extremities. A "stepping on cotton sensation" when ambulating. Varying degrees of paralysis in the upper or lower extremities. Symptoms can be contralateral and may affect all four extremities.

（4）查体颈部活动障碍或活动时有响声，并伴有疼痛或其他一些症状加重；触诊局部有疼痛和肌紧张，颈椎棘突有 2～5 个不等的病理性偏歪，棘间隙可有宽窄不一的现象，项韧带有钝厚感。

Physical examination：cervical dyskinesia or audible cracking of the neck with range of motion often times associated with pain or other symptoms. Palpatory examination：tenderness of soft tissues, muscular tension, and deviation of these cervical spines is in processes C2 through C5. Differences in width of the intraspinal spaces and dull-thick sensation of the nuchal ligaments may be found.

（5）神经根受刺激时椎间孔压缩试验、臂丛牵拉试验呈阳性，椎动脉受刺激时位置性眩晕试验呈阳性。

Positive intravertebral foramen compression test and eaten test when the nerve root is irritated. Positive positional vertigo test when vertebral artery is irritated.

（6）X 射线片可显示颈椎生理弧度改变、颈椎骨质增生、椎间隙变窄、项韧带钙化等表现。

X-ray signs：Straightening of lordosis, bony spurs and loss of intravertebral disk height, calcification of the nuchal ligaments.

（7）CT 和 MRI 可显示病变部位椎间盘突出及其与颈脊髓和神经根的关系。

CT and MRI findings：Visible intravertebral disc protrusion pushing against the cervical spinal cord and exiting nerves roots in the area of the lesions.

【小针刀治疗】Acupotomy therapy

1.1 治疗原则 Principles

针刀整体松解枕部、项部软组织的粘连、瘢痕、挛缩组织，恢复颈段软组织的力学平衡；通过调节颈段软组织的力学平衡，纠正颈椎骨关节的移位，从而解除颈部神经血管或脊髓的压迫。

Acupotomy therapy when performed integrated can sever and detach adhesions, relieve muscle spasms and decompress contracted tissues intercal to the occiput and base of the skull and in the cervical region. This process can adjust dynamic balance of the cervical soft tissues, potentiate the realignment of cervical vertebral facet joints and also can release pressure and compressed nerves, blood vessels and the cervical spinal cord.

1.2 操作方法 Procedure

(1) 体位：患者取坐位，头颈屈曲靠于椅背上（图 2-1）。

Posture：Patient is placed in the sitting position with the head and neck flexed forward and leaned on a chair back (Figure 2-1).

(2) 定点：可根据病变部位，选择以下进针点（图 2-2）。

Location：Insertion points are located according to the lesion location as follows (Figure 2-2).

①上项线以枕骨粗隆为中点，正中线旁开 2.5 cm 定两点，再向两侧旁开 5 cm 定两点。

On the line of the lineae nuchae superior, there are two points located 2.5 cm lateral of the midpoint of the external occipital protrude protuberance (the INION) bilaterally. Two further points are located 5 cm lateral to the midpoint.

18

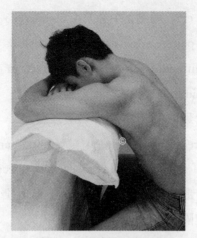

图 2 - 1 颈部治疗体位

Figure 2 - 1 Posture for neck

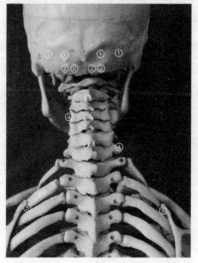

图 2 - 2 颈椎进针定点

Figure 2 - 2 Inserting points for cervical vertebrae

①上项线进针点 Inserting points on the Lineae Nuchae superior；②下项线下 2 cm 进针点 Inserting points on 2 cm below the Lineae Nuchae superior；③棘突顶点 The superior portion of the spinous processes；④颈椎横突 The transverse processes of the cervical spine；⑤肩胛提肌止点 Ending of the levitator scapulae

19

②上项线下 2 cm，两侧正中旁开 1.5 cm、2.5 cm 各定两点。

Two further points are located 2 cm below the lineae nuchae superior，two additional points are located 1.5 cm and 2.5 cm lateral to the posterior midline on each side.

③第二至第七颈椎（C2～C7），棘突顶点。

For the processes C2 through C7 points are located on the superior portion of the spinous processes of each cervical vertebra.

④颈椎横突：颞骨乳突与锁骨连线上，从乳突斜下 2 cm 处为寰椎横突，然后每间隔 1.5 cm 为下一位颈椎横突。

Additional points of the cervical spine are located along the transverse processes of each of the cervical vertebrae. The transverse process of the Atlas is located 2 cm posterior and inferior to the tip of the mastoid process of the mastoid bone bilaterally. Additional points are located following the transverse processes 1.5 cm apart following the line from the tip of the mastoid process to the clavicle.

⑤肩胛提肌止点——肩胛骨内上角。

Location of the points for the levator scapulae is located at the superior angle of each scapula.

将选定的治疗点用记号笔标明。

Mark all selected points with a marker.

（3）术野常规消毒，铺巾。

Disinfecting and draping of sterile areas should be performed in the usual fashion with anti-septics.

（4）针具：Ⅰ型 4 号针刀。

Acupotomy：type Ⅰ-4 acupotomy.

（5）针刀操作。

Manipulation of acupotomy.

①枕外隆凸上项线及上项线、下项线之间，刀口线与人体纵轴一致，针刀体向脚侧倾斜 45°，与枕骨骨面垂直，严格按照四步操作规程进针刀。针刀经皮肤、皮下组织、项筋膜达枕骨骨面后，纵疏横剥 3 刀，然后调转刀口线 90°，向下切 3 刀，范围 0.5 cm。再提针刀于皮下组织，向左右呈 45°贴枕骨向下切 3 刀，范围 0.5 cm，以松解斜方肌起点和头半棘肌止点。

Identify the Suboccipital protuberance (Inion) and region between the Nuchal Lineae superior and inferior. The body of the needle must be the same as the sagittal plane of the body access. Following the Four Steps of Acupotomy Operation Instructions, blade insertion should be oriented obliquely with the body approximately 45° caudal (downward toward the foot) and perpendicular to the surface of theoccipital bone. The Clinician inserts the acupotomy blade/needle through the skin and subcutaneous tissues extending downward to the fascia then rotates the blade/needle 90° cutting downward three small steps within half (0.5) centimeters to release the affected muscle fibers of the trapezius and semispinalis capitis muscles.

②棘突顶点，刀口线与人体纵轴一致，针刀体向头侧倾斜 45°，与棘突呈 60°，针刀经皮肤、皮下组织、项筋膜达颈椎棘突顶点骨面后，纵疏横剥；然后将针刀体逐渐向脚侧倾斜与颈椎棘突走行方向一致，调转刀口线 90°，沿棘突上缘向深部 0.5 cm 切 2 刀，宽 0.5 cm，以切开棘间韧带。

Acupotomy blade insertion of the tip of spinal processes: Direction of the needle must be the same as the central body axis. The acupotomy blade/needle is oriented in an oblique fashion 45° with the body of the blade pointed cephalad and obliquely 60° in reference to tip of the spinal process. Penetrating the skin and subcutaneous tissue in the surface of tip of spinal process, practitioner performs dredging length wise and broad wise, and then moves the needle obliquely towards the foot. The needle should be pointed the same direction as the spinous process then rotate the needle 90° to cutting downward two times along the superior border of the spinal process using to precise movements of approximately 0. 5 cm in depth and 0. 5 cm wide and live to release the affected interspinal ligaments.

③肩胛提肌止点，刀口线方向与脊柱纵轴平行，针刀体和颈部皮肤垂直，严格按照四步操作规程进针刀。针刀经皮肤、皮下组织、筋膜肌肉达肩胛骨内上角骨面，调转刀口线90°，向肩胛骨内上角边缘切3刀，范围0. 5 cm。

Strictly following the Four Steps of Acupotomy Operation Instructions, with the edge line direction of the acupotomy being parallel to the spinal axis and the body of the acupotomy being perpendicular to the skin of the neck, a practitioner inserts an acupotomy at the ending of the levator scapulae, through the skin, subcutaneous tissue, fascia and muscle to the bone surface of the interior and superior angle of the scapula, and then turns the acupotomy 90 degrees to perform a three-cut along the edge of the interior and superior angle of the scapula within 0. 5 cm in length.

④横突：刀口线与颈椎纵轴平行，针体垂直于横突前结节或后结节骨面刺入，针刀刀刃在前结节或后结节骨面上切割几下，然后将刀口沿前斜角肌纤维的方向垂直切割。

Transverse process of the affected segment: Following the edge line of the transverse process directing the needle along the cervical vertebrae axis, with the blade orientation of the blade should be perpendicular to the anterior or posterior tubercle of the transverse process. Using acupotomy technique advance the needle to the surface of the targeted tubercle and make serval small cuts perpendicular along the fibers of the anterior scalene muscle.

术毕，拔出针刀，局部压迫止血 3 分钟后，用创可贴覆盖针眼。

When acupotomy treatment finished, practitioner withdraws the acupotomy and applies pressure to the treated points for three minutes and adhesive dressing such as a Band-Aid.

（6）针刀术后手法治疗。

Manual manipulation.

首先嘱患者仰卧位，施术者正对患者头顶，用手随颈部的活动施捏按揉法；然后一只手托住患者枕部，另一只手托其下颌部，稍用力牵引，向托下颌手一侧旋转，并轻轻提拉，将错位的小关节复位。用力不能过大，以免造成新的损伤；最后提拿两侧肩部，并搓患者肩部至前臂反复 3 次（图 2 - 3）。

With the patient lying in a supine position, the practitioner is seated at the head of the patient. Using a rubbing and pinching motion massage the dorsal aspect of the neck. Holding the patient's head in one hand, cupping the patients chin with the palm of the free hand, then rotating the head and neck to one side (Usually opposite of the affected/treated side). Applying mild traction cephalad rotate and gently lifting the head quickly in the opposite direction. This maneuver may allow for relocating the facet joints of the vertebrae. The manipulation should be to avoid secondary injury to the patient. The practitioner then using pinching motion and lifting the shoulders massage the upper extremities from the shoulders to forearms repeating this process at least three times (Figure 2 - 3).

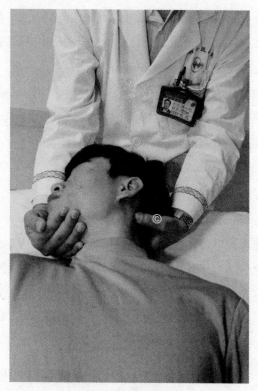

图 2 - 3　颈椎手法

Figure 2 - 3　Manual manipulation for cervical vertebrae

（由美国亚历桑那州凤凰城印地安医疗中心的杰拉德·哈里斯博士审校）

（Revised & proofed by Dr. Gerald B. Harris，II L. L. C.，Phoenix Indian Medical Center，USA）

2　枕大神经卡压症　Greater Occipital Nerve Entrapment Syndrome

【概述】Overview

　　枕大神经卡压症（GONES）是由于外伤、劳损或炎性刺激等原因导致局部软组织渗出、粘连和痉挛，刺激、卡压或牵拉枕大神经，引起头枕顶部放射痛为主要表现的一种临床常见病。

　　枕大神经在枕骨部紧贴枕骨穿出斜方肌和深筋膜，常因颈部活动、外邪侵袭等原因使局部筋伤致肌肉痉挛、深筋膜肥厚，出现炎症而产生粘连、瘢痕、挛缩，引起神经卡压而引发临床症状。

Greater Occipital Nerve Entrapment Syndrome（GONES）is commonly encountered disease caused by trauma, strain or inflammation stimulated. Tissue in certain parts of the body was excaudate, adhered, entrapped or strained in such syndrome, leading to radiated pain in occipital nerve.

Nerve clinging to occipital bone passes through the trapezius muscle and deep fascia, which usually suffered from muscle spasm and deep fascia hypertrophy attributed to neck movement and invasion of exogenous evil; such disorder will lead to inflammation induced adhesion, cicatrix and contracture, causing Nerve Entrapment and related clinical symptoms.

【诊断要点】Keys to diagnosis

　　（1）长期低头伏案工作，有颈肩部受凉史。

Patients work in bow desk and suffered cold in neck and shoulder.

（2）常表现为头枕顶部放射痛，颈肌紧张强迫头位，风池穴处有压痛。

Frequent radiated occipital pain，forced head position caused by strain in neck and shoulder，tenderness in Fengchi point.

（3）触诊可见颈第二颈椎（C2）棘突偏歪。

Tilt was found in C2 spinal process by palpation.

（4）多数患者颈椎 X 射线检查见寰枢椎旋转移位的征象（寰枢关节侧方间隙不等宽）。

X-ray inspection showed sign of atlantoaxial rotatory displacement（unequal width in atlantoaxial lateral clearance）.

【小针刀治疗】Acupotomy therapy

（1）体位：俯卧位（图 2 - 4）。

Posture：Prone position（Figure 2 - 4）.

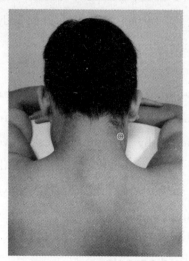

图 2 - 4　枕部治疗体位

Figure 2 - 4　Posture for occipital area

（2）定位：枕外隆凸与乳突连线的内 1/3 处（图 2-5）。将选定的治疗点用记号笔标明。

Pointing the treatment part in 1/3 of connection line between occipital spine and mastoid (Figure 2-5).

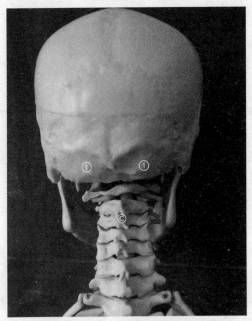

图 2-5 枕大神经进针定点

Figure 2-5 Inserting points for occipital nerve

①枕大神经进针定点 Inserting points for occipital nerve

（3）术野常规消毒，铺巾。

Disinfecting and draping in treatmental area as usual.

（4）针具：Ⅰ型 4 号直形针刀。

Instrument type：TypeⅠ-4. Straight needle blade.

（5）针刀操作：刀口线与人体纵轴一致，与枕骨垂直。刀体向脚侧倾斜 45°进针，到达上项线骨面后，调转刀口线 90°，在 0.5 cm 的范围内切 2～3 刀，松解枕大神经穿出皮下的卡压处，出针，按压针眼 3～5 分钟。

Acupotomy operation: Cutting line being paralleled with ordinate of the body, and vertical to occipital bone, inserting 45° toward the feet, when reaching the upper line of bone surface, turn the cutting line 90° and pinch spalling by 2～3 cuts within 0. 5 cm area to relieve compression caused by occipital nerve passing through subcutaneous tissue. After cutting, withdraw the acupotomy and press the points for 3～5 minutes.

注意：松解时针刀体应向脚侧倾斜，与枕骨面垂直而不是与人体纵轴线垂直，以防止刺伤椎管。

Attention: Blade should cling to the feet side when relieving, and being vertical to occipital bone instead of ordinate of the body. Such operation can be regarded as a prevention of pricking spinal canal.

（6）针刀术后手法治疗：给予手法调整治疗，患者取俯卧位，助手牵拉其双侧肩部，术者正对患者头顶站立，左肘关节屈曲，托住患者下颌，右手前臂尺侧压住患者枕骨，随颈部的活动施揉按法，然后提拿两侧肩部，并从患者肩至前臂反复揉搓几次（图 2-6）。

Postoperative treatment by maneuver: For maneuver treatment, patient was put in a prone position, with both parts of the shoulder dragged by assistant, operator standing face to vertex of the patient, with submaxilla lifted using a bent posture of the left elbow, and the right forearm ulnar pressing patient's occipital bone, rubbing along with the movement of the neck, followed by lifting both side of the shoulders, and repetitively rubbing patient from shoulder to forearm.

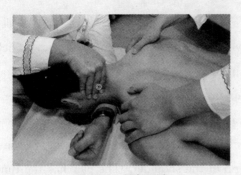

图 2-6　枕部手法

Figure 2-6　Manual manipulation for occipital area

3　肩胛提肌损伤　Injuries in Scapula Levator Muscle

【概述】Overview

肩胛提肌损伤是一种临床常见病，但大部分被诊断为颈部损伤、背部痛或颈椎病、肩周炎等，主要表现为颈部一侧及肩胛部酸胀疲乏，有重压感，多于劳累、外感受凉时症状加重。

Scapula levator muscle injury is a commonly encountered disease in clinical experience，while most of its diagnosis misled to neck injury，nostalgia，cervical spondylosis or adhesive capsulitis. Its main syndrome includes sore and fatigue in one side of the neck and scapula，with sense of stress，and aggravated by exertion and cold.

损伤出现在这对长肌，起自上 4 个颈椎的横突，肌纤维斜向后下稍外方，止于肩胛骨上角和肩胛骨脊柱缘的上部；肌肉上段位于胸锁乳突肌深侧，下段位于斜方肌的深面，有上提肩胛骨并使肩胛骨下回旋的作用。肩胛提肌由于某种特殊情况，要求肩胛骨迅速上提和向上内旋转，肩胛提肌突然收缩；而肩胛骨因受到多块肌肉不同方向的制约，多数情况下又不可能达到同步配合，导致肩胛提肌损伤。

The injury occurred in a pair of long muscle，which comprised of an upper part in deep of the sternocleidomastoid and a lower part in deep of the trapezius muscle，beginning from transverse processes in upper 4 cervical vertebrae，to outside diagonal back of the muscle fiber，ending in upper part between upper angle of the shoulder blade and spine margin of the shoulder. The pair has the function of lifting and downward convoluting of the shoulder blade. Such movement is a prerequisite that scapula was lifted under some particular conditions，and the sudden contraction of the scapula. Thus，the shoulder blade was restricted by muscles of various directions，and hardly reaches synchronization in most cases; injury in scapula levator muscle is usually occurred.

【诊断要点】Keys to diagnosis

（1）患者可有抬肩畸形，不时抖动肩膀，以缓解肩部不适感。当上肢后伸，令肩胛骨上提或内旋时，可使疼痛加剧或不能完成此动作。

Shoulder deformity can be observed as patients occasionally shaking shoulder to relieve their discomfort. When upper arm stretch backwards，as shoulder blade lifted or intorted，pain will be aggravated and the movement unable to complete.

（2）疼痛出现于肩胛骨内上角或在肩胛内侧缘。

Pain occurred in inner upper angle of the shoulder blade or in the inferior edge of shoulder blade.

（3）在肩胛骨内上角、肩胛骨内侧缘和第一至第四颈椎（C1～C4）横突有压痛点，肩胛骨内上角可扪及条索状筋结。

Tenderness may be found in inner upper angle and inferior edge of the shoulder blade，as well as transverse processes of C1~C4. There is a painful contracture can be touched in inner upper angle of the shoulder blade.

【小针刀治疗】Acupotomy therapy

(1) 体位：俯卧位（图 2-7）。

Posture：Prone posture（Figure 2-7）.

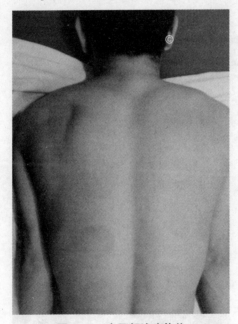

图 2-7　肩胛部治疗体位

Figure 2-7　Posture for shoulder blade

(2) 定位：

Location：

①颈椎横突后结节点：第一至第四颈椎（C1~C4）棘突间，正中旁开 2.5 cm 处，定 1~4 点。

Cervical vertebra transverse process node：In C1~C4 process,

31

2. 5 cm next to the middle，mark 1~4 points.

②肩胛骨内上角点：扪及肩胛骨内上角骨面定点。

Upper angle of the shoulder balde：Touching to mark the position on it.

③肌腹压痛点：肩胛提肌的颈根部肌腹上有硬结或条索状物上的压痛点（图 2 - 8）。

Tenderness point in muscle belly：Mark positions with callosity or ribbon shaped object in scapula muscle of the muscle belly of neck end（Figure 2 - 8）.

将选定的治疗点用记号笔标明。

Mark all selected points with a marker.

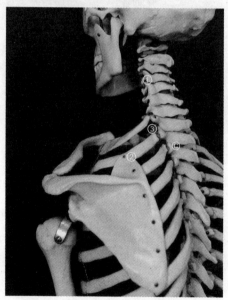

图 2 - 8　肩胛提肌进针定点

Figure 2 - 8　Inserting points for scapula elevator muscle

①颈椎横突后结节点　Cervical vertebra transverse process node；②肩胛骨内上角点　Inner upper angle of the shoulder blade；③肌腹压痛点　Tenderness point in muscle belly

（3）术野常规消毒，铺巾。

Disinfecting and draping in surgical area as usual.

（4）针具：Ⅰ型 4 号针刀。

Acupotomy：Type Ⅰ-4 acupotomy.

（5）针刀操作。

Manipulation of acupotomy.

①颈椎横突后结节点：刀口线与颈椎棘突平行，刀体与内侧皮面的夹角达 100°时，快速刺入皮肤，刀锋达关节突关节骨面上，做纵行疏通、横行剥离，针尖一定要保持在横突尖部骨面上活动。

Cervical vertebra transverse process node：Cutting line being parallel with transverse process，practitoner inserts the needle quickly at the angle of 100 degree with the inner skin surface until the edge of the needle reaching articular facet joint. Dredging lengthwise and separating broadwise with the needle tip，it must be performed on the bony surface of the transverse process.

②肩胛骨内上角点：刀口线与肩胛提肌肌纤维平行，刀体与背部皮面垂直，深达肩胛骨骨面，沿肩胛骨内上角慢慢向内侧滑动，紧贴边缘切割 3 刀。

Points in inner upper angle of the shoulder blade：Cutting line being parallel with muscle fiber of the lifting muscle in scapula，the blade body being vertical to the back of the skin，until reaching the surface of the shoulder blade，then slide inward alongside the inner upper angle，cut 3 times clinging to the margin.

③肌腹压痛点：刀口线与躯干纵轴下段呈 15°（与肌纤维方向平行），刀体与外侧面呈 60°刺入皮肤，深 1～1.5 cm，通过皮肤、皮下组织，遇到结节、条索状物和有酸胀感时，纵行疏通、横行剥离 2～3 刀。

Tenderness in muscle belly：Cutting line being 15 degree

lengthways with the lower part of the trunk (and parallel with muscle fiber), blade was inserted 60 degree with the outer surface of the skin, to the depth of 1 ∼ 1.5 cm, then pass through skin, subcutaneous tissue until reaching nodule, a strip cord like object and patients sore, followed by longitudinal deoppilant and lateral dissection for 2∼3 inserts.

术毕，拔出针刀，局部压迫止血 3 分钟后，创可贴覆盖针眼。

After treatment, withdraw the needle and press to stop bleeding for 3 minutes, then cover the points by wound plaster.

（6）针刀术后手法治疗。

Manipulation post-acupotomy treatment.

病人端坐位，让病人抬肩，施术者双手压其肩部，反复数次。再让病人患侧肩关节前屈、肘关节屈曲各 90°，放于其胸前，施术者站于其背侧，同病侧的一只手扶肩，另一只手越过病人对侧肩上，拉住病人病侧手，进行对抗牵引。用力牵拉 1∼2 次，然后让病人抬肩、屈肘扩胸，活动数次即可（图 2-9）。

Let patient sit straight and elevate shoulder, practitioner presses both sides of the shoulder repetitively. Then, the patient should bent shoulder joint forward and both elbow joint 90 degree to brace his/her chest. At the same time, practitioner is standing in the back to hold the injured side of the shoulder with one hand, while the other hand across patient's offside shoulder to drag his/her disease side shoulder for agonistic traction. After repetition for 1∼2 times, patient was instructed to elevating shoulder, bending elbow and expanding chest for several times (Figure 2-9).

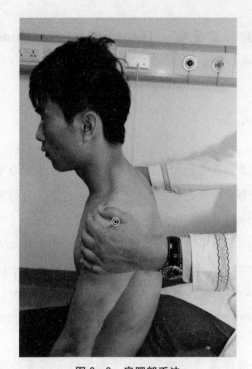

图 2-9 肩胛部手法

Figure 2-9 Manual manipulation for shoulder blade

（由美国亚历桑那州凤凰城印地安医疗中心的杰拉德·哈里斯博士校审）

（Revised & proofed by Dr. Gerald B. Harris, II L. L. C., Phoenix Indian Medical Center，USA）

4 胸椎小关节紊乱症 Disorders of the Small Joint of Thoracic Vertebra

【概述】Overview

胸椎小关节紊乱症是指胸椎小关节在外力作用下发生解剖位置的改变，引起关节囊滑膜嵌顿而形成的错缝，且不能自行复位而导致的疼痛和功能受限等症状的一种病症。

Disorders of the small joint of thoracic vertebrae are defined as a change of anatomic relation between thoracic facet joints, refered to displacement following by the joint capsule synovialinterposing. The displacement can not replace by the joint itself so as to present painful back and moto limitation.

胸椎小关节即关节突关节，由于胸椎后关节突关节面近似冠状位，两侧有肋骨支撑，胸椎的稳定性相对于颈椎和腰椎为强，发生后关节错缝的机会相对于颈椎和腰椎较少。但当突然的外力牵拉、体位变换不当，或长时间处于低头含胸坐位，使后关节不能承受所分担的应力时，则有可能引起胸椎后关节错缝病变。

The small joint of thoracic vertebrae is actually the facet joint. The articular surface of the facet joint is on a coronal position with the support by ribs on both sides. Incidence of displacement of thoracic facet joints is less than that happened in cervical vertebrae and lumbar vertebrae for stability of thoracic vertebrae being better than the one of cervical vertebrae and lumbar vertebrae. The displacement of thoracic facet joints may result in abnormal loading of facet joints by foreign force traction, improper change of posture or sitting in a head down on chest position frequently.

【诊断要点】Keys to Diagnosis

（1）有抬、扛、提、举及身体扭转等动作而致的外伤史或长期不良姿势病史。

The patient has the history of injury by lifting, carrying, turning the body, or a history of a long-term improper posture.

（2）急性损伤者，可表现为一侧或双侧胸背疼痛，疼痛可沿肋间由后向前走向及向腰腹部放射，咳嗽、深呼吸时疼痛加剧。

The symptoms and signs include unilateral or bilateral pectoralgia and backache in acute cases, which radiate along the intercostal region to the lumbo-abdominal region and become aggravated when coughing or deeply breathing.

（3）伤后病程长者多表现为背部酸痛、沉重感，每遇阴雨天或久站、久坐以及弯腰稍久均可使症状加重。

Aching pain and heavy sensation in the back occur in chronic cases. The symptoms are worsened in cloudy or wet weather, or by long standing, sitting, or long bending over.

（4）部分患者可兼有胸腹腔脏器的功能性紊乱症状，如心律失常、呼吸困难、胃脘胀闷、大便秘结等。

Functional disturbance of viscera in some cases, such as arrhythmia, dyspnea, distension and fullness in the stomach, constipation and so on.

（5）查体大部分患者活动正常，少数活动受限（尤其是后伸较明显），可有棘旁压痛、棘突病理性偏歪及邻近肌肉紧张，棘上韧带可有剥离或钝厚感。

Signs of the physical examination: normal activity in most patients, limited activity (backward extension in particular), tenderness by the spinous process and tension of the adjacent muscles, stripping or thick sensation in the supraspinal ligaments in a few patients.

（6）胸椎正侧位 X 射线平片，可有椎体退行性改变，韧带钙化及胸段脊柱代偿性侧凸或后凸畸形。

X-ray signs: retrograde change of the vertebral body, calcification of the ligaments, compensatory thoracic scoliosis or kyphosis on the anteroposterior or lateral X-rays of the thoracic spine.

【小针刀治疗】Acupotomy therapy

（1）体位：俯卧位（图 2 - 10）。

Posture: Prone position (Figure 2 - 10).

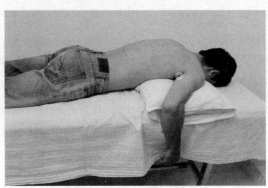

图 2 - 10　胸椎治疗体位

Figure 2 - 10　Posture for thoracic vertebrae

（2）定位（图 2 - 11）。

Location (Figure 2 - 11).

①棘突：以患椎棘突顶点为中心作为第 1 点，再在上胸椎棘突、下胸椎棘突各取 1 点。

Spinal process: Mark the first point at spinal process of lesion thoracic vertebrae, and then mark two more points in both processes above and below the first point.

②胸椎小关节：从患椎棘突顶点向两侧旁开 2 cm 各取 1 点，是胸椎小关节位置。同法在患椎上胸椎、下胸椎两侧小关节各取 2 点。

Facet joint：From the spinal process' top of affected thoracic vertebrae, mark one point 2 cm lateral the midline on each side. Mark two points for each thoracic vertebra above and below using the same method mentioned above.

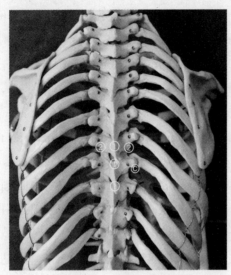

图 2 - 11 胸椎进针定点

Figure 2 - 11 Inserting points of thoracic vertebrae

①棘突 Spinal process；②胸椎小关节 Facet joint

（3）术野常规消毒，铺巾。

Disinfecting and draping in treatmental area as usual.

（4）针具：Ⅰ型 4 号直形针刀。

Acupotomy：Type Ⅰ-4 acupotomy.

（5）针刀操作。

Manipulation of acupotomy.

①胸椎棘突点：刀口线与人体纵轴一致，针刀体向头侧倾斜 45°，

与棘突呈 60°。严格按照四步操作规程进针刀。针刀经皮肤、皮下组织、筋膜达胸椎棘突顶点骨面后，纵疏横剥；然后将针刀体逐渐向脚侧倾斜与棘突走行方向一致，调转刀口线 90°，沿棘突上缘向深部 0.5 cm切 2 刀，范围 0.5 cm，以切开棘间韧带。

Spinal process of thoracic vertebrae: Edge line direction of the acupotomy must be the same as the body axis. Acupotomy is inserted 45 degrees obliquely with the body of needle upward to the head and 60 degrees to the spinal process. Strictly following Four steps of Acupotomy Operation Instructions, practitioner inserts the acupotomy to the top of spinal process through skin, subcutaneous tissue and fascia nuchae to dredge lengthwise and broadwise, then moves the needle obliquely downwards the foot, the neddle pointing the same direction as the spinal process, then turns the needle 90 degrees to cut downward along superior side of the spinal process 2 times within 0.5 cm in depth and 0.5 cm in length for releasing affected ligamenta interspinalia.

②胸椎小关节点：刀口线与人体纵轴一致，垂直进针。针刀经皮肤、皮下组织、筋膜达胸椎小关节关节囊骨面后，纵疏横剥数刀。

Facet joint of thoracic vertebrae: Edge line direction of the needle must be the same as the body axis. Practitioner inserts the acupotomy perpendicular to the bony surface of the thoracic facet joint capsule through skin, subcutaneous tissue and fascia nuchae to dredging lengthwise and seperating broadwise for several times.

（6）针刀术后手法治疗。

Manipulation post-acupotomy treatment.

患者俯卧位，双手置于体侧。施术者立于一侧，双手掌重叠置于患椎棘突部；嘱患者深吸气，待其吐气后双手向前下方约 45°推按，可听到"咯"的一声，手法完毕（图 2-12）。

Patient lying in a prone position and placing both arms beside his body, a practitioner presses the spinous process of affected vertebrae with two overlapped hands, asks patient breath-in deeply, and then makes upward push and pressure at an angle of 45 degrees to the spine at the end of patient breath-out. A sound "chuck" is often heard. Manipulation is finished (Figure 2-12).

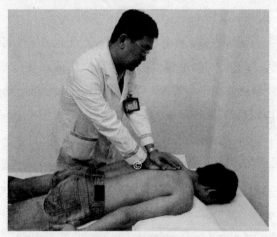

图 2-12 胸椎手法

Figure 2-12 Manual manipulation for thoracic vertebrae

（由美国亚历桑那州凤凰城印地安医疗中心的杰拉德·哈里斯博士审校）

(Revised & proofed by Dr. Gerald B. Harris, II L. L. C., Phoenix Indian Medical Center, USA)

5 急性腰椎后关节滑膜嵌顿 Acute Lumbar Facet Joint Synovial

【概述】Overview

腰椎后关节滑膜嵌顿，亦称腰椎后关节紊乱症或腰椎间小关节综合征，中医称为"闪腰"。多由轻度的急性腰扭伤或弯腰猛然起立导致，关节突扭动使滑膜嵌插于关节内，引起剧烈腰痛和脊椎活动受限。

Acute lumbar facet joint synovial is also called as disorders of lumbar facet joint or syndrome of lumbar facet joint. It is defined as "strained back" in TCM theory. Patient presents severe painful lower back and limitation of the spine movement related to synovialinterposing following by twisted processus articularis because of mild acute lumbar sprain or stand-up suddenly from a bow posture.

腰椎上关节突、下关节突的关节面互成直角，一个呈冠状位，另一个呈矢状位，活动的范围较大。当腰部突然活动，腰椎小关节后缘间隙张开，使关节内产生负压，吸入滑膜。此时，腰椎突然后伸，滑膜就可能来不及退出而被嵌夹在关节之间，形成腰椎后小关节滑膜嵌顿或小关节错位。滑膜充血水肿并刺激神经，从而引发剧烈的腰痛和运动障碍。

The articular surface of superior articular process and inferior articular process are perpendicular to each other. The first is on a coronal position and the other is on a sagittal position that allows wide-range moto for waist. When patient makes a waist movement unexpectedly, a sudden opening of the posterior interspace of lumbar facet joints produces a negative pressure which attracts the synovium, resulting in synovialinterposing or displacement of the facet joint. Affected synovium becomes hyperemia, edema and causes nerve irritation, those lead to a severe pain and limitation of movement in patient's waist.

【诊断要点】Keys to Diagnosis

（1）多有腰部扭挫伤史。伤后立即出现腰部难以忍受的剧痛，不能活动，有的疼痛可向臀部和大腿后侧放射。

Most patients have the history of sprain and contusion in the lumbar region. The symptoms and signs include lumbar dyskinesia intolerable severe pains in the lumbar region, which spear immediately after injury and transmit to the buttocks or the posterior thighs in some cases.

（2）患者呈强迫体位，腰椎生理曲度变直或后突或侧突，活动功能受限，腰过伸时疼痛加剧，腰前屈时疼痛略缓解。

The patient kept forced posture, straightened physiological curvature of the lumbar spine, or scoliosis, or kyphosis, limited activity, worsening the pains in lumbar hyperextension but easing the pains in lumbar anteflexion.

（3）查体见腰部肌肉痉挛紧张或僵硬，第四至第五腰椎（L4～L5）或第五腰椎至第一骶骨（L5～S1）棘突旁有深在性压痛点，一般无神经根刺激症状；腰椎有 2～3 个不等的病理性棘突偏歪。

Signs found in the physical examination: lumbar muscular spasm and tension or stiffness, deep-seated tenderness points beside the spinous processes of L4 and L5, or L5 and S1, no sighs of nerve root irritation, phathological deviation of 2～3 spinous processes.

（4）X 射线片显示腰椎生理曲度变直或后突或侧弯，有的可显示后关节排列紊乱或椎间隙和后关节腔左右宽窄不一的征象。

X-ray signs include straightened physiological curvature of the lumbar spine, or scoliosis, or kyphosis; disturbed arrangement of the posterior joints or unequal right-left width of the intervertebral space and the posterior articular cavity in some cases.

【小针刀治疗】Acupotomy therapy

(1) 体位：俯卧位（图 2-13）。

Posture：Prone position（Figure 2-13）.

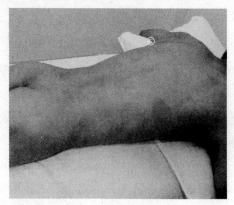

图 2-13 腰椎治疗体位

Figure 2-13 Posture for lumbal vertebrae

(2) 定位（图 2-14）。

Location（Figure 2-14）.

①腰椎小关节：根据椎旁压痛点确定病变所在腰椎，在其棘突顶点正中线旁开 2 cm，两侧各取 1 点；同法在患椎上位椎、下位椎的腰椎旁取点。

Facet joint of lumbar vertebrae：Affected vertebra segment is located according to where a pressing pain point is. From the spinal process' top of affected lumbar vertebrae, mark one point 2 cm lateral the

44

mid-line on eath side. Mark two more points for each lumbar vertebra above and below using the same method mentioned above.

②竖脊肌中部与下部：在胸腰椎交界处，正中线旁开 3 cm，两侧各取 1 点；第五腰椎（L5）棘突下方骶中嵴，向两侧旁开 2 cm 各取 1 点。

Middle section and lower section of erector muscle of spine：Mark the two points 3 cm lateral the mid-line at the juncture of thoracic vertebrae and lumbar vertebrae on each side. Mark other two points 2 cm lateral the mid-line on each side，at cristae sacralis media level which locates below the L5 spinal process.

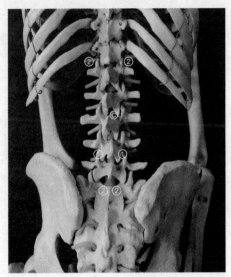

图 2 - 14　腰椎后关节进针定点

Figure 2 - 14　Inserting points for lumbar facet joint

①腰椎小关节　Facet joint of lumbar vertebrae；②竖脊肌中部与下部 Middle section and lower section of erector muscle of spine

（3）术野常规消毒，铺巾。

Disinfecting and draping in treatmental area as usual.

45

（4）针具：Ⅰ型4号直形针刀。

Acupotomy：Type Ⅰ-4 acupotomy.

（5）针刀操作。

Manipulation of acupotomy.

①小关节点：刀口线与人体纵轴一致，垂直进针。针刀经皮肤、皮下组织、肌肉达腰椎小关节关节囊骨面后，行"十"字切开，范围0.5 cm。

Facet joint of lumbar vertebrae：Edge line direction of the needle must be the same as the body axis. Practitioner inserts the acupotomy perpendicular to the bony surface of the lumbar facet joint capsule through skin，subcutaneous tissue and fascia nuchae to make a cross cut within 0.5 cm range.

②竖脊肌中部与下部：刀口线与人体纵轴一致，垂直进针，经皮肤、皮下组织到达竖脊肌，每个点上切割3刀。

Middle section and lower section of erector muscle of spine：Edge line direction of the acupotomy must be the same as the body axis. Practitioner inserts the acupotomy perpendicular to the erector muscle of spine through skin，subcutaneous tissue, and then performs a three-cut on each point.

（6）针刀术后手法治疗。

Manipulation post-acupotomy treatment.

斜扳法：

Oblique pulling manipulation：

患者侧卧，床侧下肢自然伸直，上侧下肢膝、髋关节屈曲70°～80°。施术者一肘部置于患者肩部，另一肘部置于同侧臀部，向相反方向用力推拉，当遇到阻力时，突然加大推拉力，常可听到"咯"的一声（图2-15）。

The patient in a lateral position extends the lower extremity next to the bed naturally and flexes the knee and hip of the other lower extremity at 70 to 80 degrees. The performer places one elbow in front of patient's shoulder, and the other elbow on his hip, then thrusts patient's waist in opposite directions. When the resistance appears, the push and pull are suddenly increased and a sound "chuck" is often heard (Figure 2 - 15).

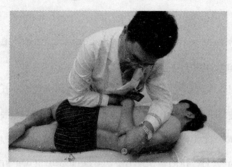

图 2 - 15 腰椎手法

Figure 2 - 15 Manual manipulation for lumbal vertebrae

6 腰椎间盘突出症 Lumbar Disc Herniation

【概述】Overview

腰椎间盘突出症是由于腰椎间盘纤维环破裂，髓核从破裂处突出于后方或椎管内，腰椎神经遭受刺激或压迫而引起的以腰部疼痛，一侧下肢或双侧下肢麻木、疼痛为主要临床表现的一种病症。本病男性多发于女性，临床上第四腰椎至第五腰椎（L4～L5）、第五腰椎至第一骶骨间（L5～S1）发病率较高，约占总数的 95％。发病的外因是外伤、劳损和寒湿侵袭等，内因是椎间盘的退行性改变。

Protrusion of the lumbar intervertebral disc is a kind of disease resulted from rupture of lumbar annulus, and the nucleus pulposus protruding into the rear of spinal canal. So lumbar nerves suffer from irritating or compressing and caused the waist pain, unilateral or bilateral lower limb pain and numbness as the main clinical manifestations. Male suffer from the disease more than female. Clinically, L4~L5 or L5~S1 was in a high incidence, accounting for about 95% of the total. Endogenous pathogenic factor is disk degeneration, while exogenous pathogenic factors include trauma, strain and impingement of pathogenic cold and wet.

外伤与劳损：腰部活动主要依靠腰椎周围肌肉，长期弯腰、负重或坐位工作会使肌肉肌腱等软组织外伤或劳损，引发腰椎失稳。

Trauma and strain: Waist movement depends on muscles around lumbar vertebrae. By body bowing, overloading or siting for a long period of time, soft tissue injury and strain involving muscles and tendons result in lumbar vertebrae instability.

寒湿侵袭：长期在寒冷、潮湿环境下工作、生活，寒湿之邪侵袭经脉，可阻遏经气运行，引发腰部痹痛、活动不利。

Impingement of pathogenic cold and wet: Working or living often in a cold or wet condition, lower back pain and moto limitation resulted from Qi fluidity failure of the meridians caused by impingement of pathogenic cold and wet.

椎间盘退变：椎间盘退变始于纤维环后外侧撕裂，髓核水分和蛋白多糖的丢失使间盘高度降低。椎间盘突出带来的疼痛可因神经根直接受压或髓核退行性变的碎片引起，或因自身免疫反应所致。

Disc degeneration: Disc degeneration starts with tears in the posterolateral region of the annulus. The subsequent loss of water content and proteoglycans in the nucleus then leads to a decrease of disc height. The pain accompanying disc herniation may be caused by direct pressure on the nerve root or may be induced by breakdown products from a degenerated nucleus pulposus or by an autoimmune reaction.

【诊断要点】Keys to Diagnosis

（1）大多数患者有腰部急性、慢性外伤史。

Most patients have the history of acute or chronic injury in the lumbar region.

（2）腰痛伴向一侧下肢放射性疼痛或向双侧下肢放射性疼痛麻木。

Symptoms and signs include lumbago with pains radiation to lower extremity or with pains and numbness in both lower extremities.

（3）腹压增加时疼痛加剧，如咳嗽、打喷嚏时。

Pain gets worse when abdominal pressure increasing such as coughing or sneezing.

（4）棘突间旁有压痛与放射痛；腰椎有 2～3 个不等的病理性棘突偏歪；患椎上下的棘上韧带有索状剥离滑动感，伴有压痛；患椎上棘间隙、下棘间隙有宽窄不一的征象。

Tenderness and radiating pains about the interspinal region; pathological deviation of two or three spinous processes; cord-like stripping and sliding sensation with tenderness in the supraspinal ligaments above and below the affected vertebrae; unequal widths of the interspinal spaces above and below the affected vertebrae.

（5）直腿抬高试验及加强试验呈阳性。

Positive straight-leg-raising and intensive straight-leg-raising tests.

（6）仰卧挺腹试验、颈静脉压迫试验、抬颈压胸试验均为阳性。

Positive results of supine-position abdomen-raising test，Queckenstedt's test，neck-raising and chest-pressing tests.

（7）趾背伸试验患侧减弱；早期痛觉过敏，稍后则减退。

There are attenuated myodynamia on the affected side in toe dorsal extension test，hyperalgesia at early stage and hypoalgesia afterwards.

（8）腰肌痉挛，脊柱畸形和活动受限。

Lumbar muscles are spasm，deformity and limited activity of the spine.

（9）X射线片示：脊椎侧凸，前凸消失，椎间隙变窄，椎缘增生。

X-ray signs：Scoliosis，loss of lordosis，narrowed intervertbra space，hyperplasia of vertebral edge.

（10）CT、MRI检查可清楚显示椎间盘突出的部位、大小、形态和神经根、硬膜囊受压移位的征象。

CT or MRI shows clear findings of the site，size and shape of the intervertebral disc hernia，displacement of nerve root and dura due to compression.

【小针刀治疗】Acupotomy therapy

（1）体位：俯卧位（图 2 - 16）。

Posture：Prone position（Figure 2 - 16）.

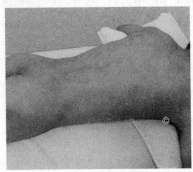

图 2 - 16 腰椎治疗体位

Figure 2 - 16   Posture for lumbal vertebrae

（2）定位：以第四至第五腰椎（L4～L5）椎间盘突出为例（图2-17）。

Location：Taking L4～L5 intervertebral disc protrusion as an example（Figure 2-17）.

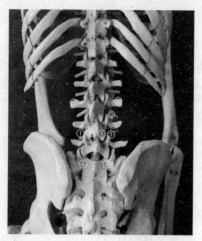

图 2-17　腰椎间盘突出症进针定点

Figure 2-17　Inserting points for prolapse of lumar intervertebral disc

①腰椎小关节点　Facet joint of lumbar vertebrae；②第三腰椎横突点　L3 transverse process；③第四至第五腰椎棘间韧带点　L4～L5 ligamenta interspinalia；④竖脊肌起点　Erector spinae

①腰椎小关节点：第四腰椎（L4）棘突和第五腰椎（L5）棘突最高点水平，正中线旁分别开 1 cm、2 cm，即小关节内侧、外侧，两侧各取 2 点。

Facet joint of lumbar vertebrae：On top of spinal processes of L4 and L5，mark two points 1 cm lateral and 2 cm lateral the midline on each side. Those points autruely locate at interior side and exterior side of the facet joint.

②第三腰椎（L3）横突点：第二至第三腰椎（L2～L3）棘间隙，正中线旁开 3 cm，两侧各取 1 点。

L3 transverse process：Between L2～L3 spinal processes，mark one point 3 cm lateral the midline on each side.

③第四至第五腰椎（L4～L5）棘间韧带点：第五腰椎（L5）棘突顶点，后正中线上。

L4～L5 ligamenta interspinalia：Chose one point on the top of L5 spinal process in the midline posterior.

④竖脊肌起点：第五腰椎（L5）棘突下方骶中嵴，中线旁开 2 cm 各取 1 点。

Erector spinae：Mark two points 2 cm lateral the midline on each side，at cristae sacralis media level which locates below L5 spinal process.

（3）术野常规消毒，铺巾。

Disinfecting and draping in treatmental area as usual.

（4）针具：Ⅰ型 4 号直形针刀。

Acupotomy：Type Ⅰ-4 acupotomy.

（5）针刀操作。

Manipulation of acupotomy.

①腰椎小关节点：刀口线与人体纵轴一致，垂直进针。针刀经皮肤、皮下组织、肌肉达腰椎小关节关节囊骨面后，行"十"字切开，范围 0.5 cm。

Facet joint of lumbar vertebrae：Edge line direction of the acupotomy must be the same as the body axis. Practitioner inserts the acupotomy perpendicular to the bony surface of the lumbar facet joint capsule through skin，subcutaneous tissue and fascia nuchae to make a cross cut within 0.5 cm range.

②第三腰椎（L3）横突点：刀口线与人体纵轴一致，垂直进针，针刀尖落在横突骨面后，再向外移动针尖至横突尖部，向深部 0.5 cm 处刺数下。

L3 transverse process：Edge line direction of the acupotomy must be the same as the body axis. Practitioner inserts the acupotomy perpendicular to the bony surface of the transverse process through skin，subcutaneous tissue and turns the needle tip outward to touch tip of the transverse process，and cuts several times within 0.5 cm in depth.

③第四至第五腰椎（L4～L5）棘间韧带点：针刀体与皮肤垂直，从第五腰椎（L5）棘突顶点进针刀，刀口线与脊柱纵轴平行，针刀经皮肤、皮下组织直达棘突骨面，贴棘突上缘斜刺，深度约0.5 cm；再向棘突下缘斜刺，深度约0.5 cm；最后贴骨面向棘突两侧分别用提插刀法切割3刀，深度约0.5 cm。

L4 ～ L5 ligamenta interspinalia：Edge line direction of the acupotomy must be the same as the body axis. Acupotomy is inserted perpendicular to the top of L5 spinal process through skin，subcutaneous tissue. Practitioner turns the needle tip upward to superior side of the spinal process within 0.5 cm in depth，and then turns the needle tip downward to inferior side of the spinal process within 0.5 cm in depth，at last turns the needle tip to both side of the spinal process within 0.5 cm in depth to perform a three-cut with lifting-thrusting method.

注意：不能深刺至黄韧带，以免刺入椎管内。

Attention：Acupotomy must not be inserted to ligamentum flavum to avoid punching in spinal canal.

④竖脊肌起点：刀口线与人体纵轴一致，垂直进针，经皮肤、皮下组织到达竖脊肌，每个点上切割3刀。

Erector spinae：Edge line direction of the acupotomy must be the same as the body axis. Practitioner inserts the acupotomy perpendicular to the erector muscle of spine through skin， subcutaneous tissue, and then performs a three-cut on each point.

（6）针刀术后手法治疗。

Manipulation post-acupotomy treatment.

①斜扳法：见"急性腰椎后关节滑膜嵌顿"中的"斜扳法"（第46页）（图 2 - 18）。

Oblique pulling manipulation: Please refer to the chapter "Acute Lumbar Facet Joint Synovial" (Figure 2 - 18).

②直腿抬高加压法：施术者将患者患侧下肢伸直，慢慢抬高，并按压其足底使踝关节背伸。

Straight leg-raising manipulation: Practitioner rases patient's affected leg with the leg being straight envently, and then pushes patient's ankle joint upward.

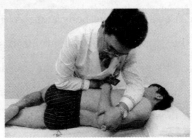

图 2 - 18　腰椎手法

Figure 2 - 18　Manual manipulation for lumbal vertebrae

7　第三腰椎横突综合征　Syndrome of the Third Lumbar Transverse Process

【概述】Overview

第三腰椎横突综合征是由第三腰椎横突附着点的肌肉、韧带损伤所致的腰痛，多见于成年体力劳动者。

Syndrome of the third lumbar transverse process, being common in the adult manual workers, shows lower back pain which is caused by muscle and ligament injury at their attachment points to the transverse processes.

第三腰椎（L3）横突特别长，且水平位伸出，附近有血管、神经束经过，有较多的肌筋膜附着。第三腰椎处于腰椎生理前凸弧度的顶点，为承受力学传递的重要部位，因此易受外力作用的影响，容易受损伤而引起该处附着肌肉撕裂、出血、瘢痕粘连、筋膜增厚挛缩，使血管神经束受摩擦、刺激和压迫而产生症状。

L3 transverse processes are especially longer than those of others and protrude in a horizontal position. There are blood vessels and nerves passing the processes area. Many muscles and fascia muscularis adhere to the process, too. Located in the top of lumbar vertebral physiological curvature, L3 bears mechanical transmission and overload injury leading to muscles tear, bleeding, contracture, adhesion, and fascia thicken and cicatrice. Symptoms indicate friction, irritation and compression of blood vessels and nerve bunch around the transverse processes.

【诊断要点】Keys to diagnosis

（1）腰部有劳损史。

The patient has the history of injury in the lumbar region.

（2）腰部一侧或双侧疼痛，活动受限，可有向臀部或大腿外侧放射性疼痛，疼痛与腹压增加无关。

The symptoms and signs include limited activity, pains on one or both sides of the lumbar region. The pain radiates to the buttocks or to the lateral thigh but the pain is not related to abdominal pressure increasing.

（3）患侧腰肌紧张、僵硬，于第三腰椎（L3）横突尖端可触及结节状硬结，压痛明显，第二至第三腰椎（L2～L3）棘突可有病理性偏歪。

Tension and stiffness of the lumbar muscles on the affected side，palpable nodular induration and obvious tenderness on the top of L3 transverse process，and pathological deviation of the spinous processes of L2 and L3.

（4）直腿抬高试验呈阳性，但直腿抬高加强试验、"4"字试验呈阴性。

Positive straight-leg-raising test but negative intensive straight-leg-raising and Patrick's test.

（5）X射线片可见第三腰椎（L3）横突过长或粗大。

X-ray signs show longer or bigger L3 transverse process.

【小针刀治疗】Acupotomy therapy

（1）体位：俯卧位（图 2 - 19）。

Posture：Prone position （Figure 2 - 19）.

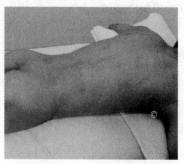

图 2 - 19　腰椎治疗体位

Figure 2 - 19　Posture for lumbal vertebrae

（2）定点：第三腰椎（L3）横突点，第二至第三腰椎（L2～L3）棘突间，正中线旁开 3 cm，患侧取 1 点（图 2 - 20）。

Location：L3 transverse process：Between L2 ～ L3 spinal processes，mark one point 3 cm lateral the midline on effected side (Figure 2 - 20).

（3）术野常规消毒，铺巾。

Disinfecting and draping in surgical area as usual.

（4）针具：Ⅰ型 4 号针刀。

Acupotomy：Type Ⅰ-4 acupotomy.

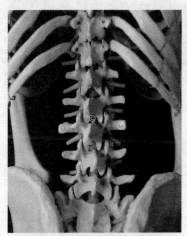

图 2 - 20　第三腰椎横突进针定点

Figure 2 - 20　Inserting points for syndrome of L3 transverse

①L3 横突点　L3 transverse process

（5）针刀操作。

Manipulation of acupotomy.

刀口线与人体纵轴一致，垂直进针，针刀尖落在横突骨面后，再向外移动针尖至横突尖部，向深部 0.5 cm 处刺数下。

Edge line direction of the acupotomy must be the same as the body axis. Practitioner inserts the acupotomy perpendicular to the bony surface of the transverse process through skin, subcutaneous tissue and turns the needle tip outward to touch tip of the transverse process, and cuts several times within 0.5 cm in depth.

注意：进针时必须先找到横突骨面再向横突尖部移动；针刺横突尖部位要紧贴横突尖部骨面，不可深入，以防小针刀刺入腹腔。

Attention：Insertion must be touched the bony surface of the transverse process first and be moved to tip of the process. Practitioner must keep the needle tip closely against the tip of transverse process to avoid inserting deeper into abdominal cavity.

（6）针刀术后手法治疗。

Manipulation after acupotomy treatment.

斜扳法：见"急性腰椎后关节滑膜嵌顿"中的"斜扳法"（第46页）（图2-21）。

Oblique pulling manipulation：Please refer to the chapter "Acute Lumbar Facet Joint Synovial"（Figure 2-21）.

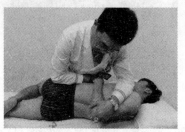

图 2-21　腰椎手法

Figure 2-21　Manual manipulation for lumbal vertebrae

8　腰椎椎管狭窄症　Stenosis of the Lumbar Spine

【概述】 Overview

腰椎椎管狭窄症临床表现呈多样性，以腰痛和下肢功能障碍为主诉，由发育性和继发性椎管、神经根管或椎间孔狭窄，引起神经组织受压。

Stenosis of the lumbar spine is a clinical entity that is responsible for a variety of complaints ranging from low back pain to lower-extremity dysfunction. The condition has been defined as any developmental or acquired narrowing of the spinal canal, nerve root canals, or intervertebral foramina that result in compressing of neural elements.

生理性的狭窄随年龄增长而出现。椎管容积因屈曲而增大，但随伸展而变小；椎管狭窄可因前方椎间盘突出、后方的黄韧带肥厚或小关节突关节侵占而进一步发展。椎间盘退行性变引起小关节压力增加，从而使小关节及邻近组织发生炎症和肥大，并最终累及椎管。由于椎管容积的变小以缓慢和渐进的方式出现，以致多数患者的神经组织逐渐适应，因此尽管病人已经存在退行性狭窄，但很少人会突然出现临床症状。

Some physiologic narrowing of the canal occurs with age. The canal volume increases in flexion and decreases in extension. Narrowing of the spinal canal can further occur by bulging of the disk anteriorly, by buckling of the ligamentum flavum posteriorly, and by encroachment of the articular facets. Degeneration of the intervertebral disk causes increased stress on the facet joint and can lead to arthrosis and hypertrophy of facets and adjacent strctures. This will ultimately compromise the spinal canal. The decrease in canal volume occurs at such a slow and gradual pace that the neurologic structures in most patients accommodate to it, with the result that there may be surprisingly few neurologic symptoms even in patients with advanced degenerative stenosis.

椎管狭窄的患者经历疼痛的原因很复杂，可归纳为机械性、缺血性、炎症性和其他多种因素。最直接的因素是脊髓和毗邻神经根部的单纯机械性压迫。根据神经化学理论，神经纤维因营养小血管的压迫而失营养。硬脊膜及神经根出口的炎症状态有同样意义。

The cause of pain experienced by patients with stenosis is perplexing and has been attributed to mechanical, ischemic, inflammatory, and various other mechanisms. The simplest explanation, of couse, is pure mechanical compression of cord and adjacent roots. According to the neurois chemic explanation, the nerve fibers are nutritionally deprived by compression of the small nutrient vessels. Inflammatory conditions of the dura and exiting nerve root are equally suspect.

椎管狭窄症分为先天性和继发性，狭窄的部位分为中央型和侧方型。中央型的狭窄肥大结构对脊髓产生圆周形压力；侧方型狭窄与椎间孔变窄有关，因而将其分为三个区域，即入口区、中间区和出口区。

Spinal stenosis is classified as congenital or acquired. The location of stenosis can be central or lateral. In central stenosis, hypertrophied structures cause circumferential pressure of the spinal cord. Lateral stenosis is associated with narrowing of the foraminal canal, which is devided into three separated zones: the entrance zone, the middle zone, and the exit zone.

【诊断要点】Keys to Diagnosis

退行性椎管狭窄症首发于年长者，男性比女性多见，对下腰段影响最严重。临床表现多样化，在许多病例中，有隐性发病和缓慢进展的腰痛、臀部痛和大腿痛。疼痛是弥散而不是节段性和片段性的，几乎所有的患者报告下肢痛可因体位改变而改变，疼痛一般出现在站立或行走，休息、躺下、坐下或采用弯腰位置后减轻，这种症状称为间歇性跛行。

In degenerative spinal stenosis, which occurs primarily in elderly individuals and is seen more commonly in men than in women, the lower lumbar segments are affected the most severely. The pattern of complaints varies among patients. In many cases, there is an insidious onset and low progression of pain in the lower back, buttock and thigh. The pain is generally diffused rather than neurosegmental and is episodic. Nearly all patients report that their lower extremity pain is altered by changes in position. It generally occurs with standing or walking and is relieved by rest, lying, sitting, or adopting a position of flexion at the waist. This is the hallmark symptom of pseudoclaudication.

【影像学分析】Imaging studies

平片中可见椎间盘退行性改变、小关节骨关节炎、椎体前滑脱、前后位片上椎弓根距离变窄。CT 能准确测定椎管内径，硬膜囊前后径小于 10 mm，必然与椎管狭窄的临床发现有关联。MRI 对于确认椎管狭窄症比 CT 扫描而言，对比度更明显。

Findings on plain radiographs include degenerative disk disease, osteoarthritis of the facets，spondylolisthesis，and narrowing of the interpedicular distance as seen on the anteroposterior view. CT scanning，which is now commonly used to evaluate the spinal elements，allows for accurate measurement of the canal dimensions. A dural sac with an anteroposterior diameter of less than 10 mm is correlates with clinical findings of stenosis. MRI is comparable to contrast-enhanced CT scanning in its ability to demonstrate spinal stenosis.

【小针刀治疗】Acupotomy therapy

(1) 体位：俯卧位（图 2 - 22）。

Posture：Prone position（Figure 2 - 22）.

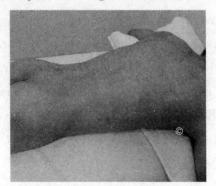

图 2 - 22　腰椎治疗体位

Figure 2 - 22　Posture for lumbal vertebrae

(2) 定位（图 2 - 23）。

Location（Figure 2 - 23）. ·

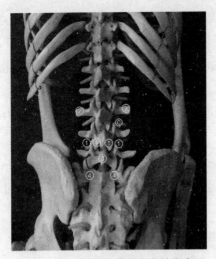

图 2 - 23 腰椎管狭窄症进针定点

Figure 2 - 23 Inserting points for stenosis of the lumbar spine

①腰椎小关节点 Facet joint of lumbar vertebrae；②L3 横突点 L3 transverse process；③L4～L5、L5～S1 棘间韧带点 L4～L5 and L5～S1 ligamentas interspinalia；④竖脊肌起点 Erector spinae

①腰椎小关节点：第四腰椎（L4）棘突和第五腰椎（L5）棘突最高点水平，正中线旁分别开 1 cm、2 cm，即小关节内侧、外侧，两侧各取 2 点。

Facet joint of lumbar vertebrae：On the top of spinal processes of L4 and L5，mark two points 1 cm lateral and 2 cm lateral the midline on each side. Those points locate at interior side and exterior side of the facet joint.

②L3 横突点：第二至第三腰椎（L2～L3）棘间隙，正中线旁开 3 cm，两侧各取 1 点。

L3 transverse process：Between L2～L3 spinal processes，mark one point 3 cm lateral the midline on each side.

③第四至第五腰椎（L4～L5）、第五腰椎至第一骶骨（L5～S1）棘

63

间韧带点：第五腰椎（L5）和第一骶骨（S1）棘突顶点，后正中线上。

L4～L5 and L5～S1 ligamentas interspinalia：Two points on the top of L5 and S1 spinal process in the midline posteriorly will be chosen.

④竖脊肌起点：第五腰椎（L5）棘突下方骶中嵴，中线旁开 2 cm，各取 1 点。

Erector spinae：Mark two points 2 cm lateral the midline on each side，at cristae sacralis media level which locates below the L5 spinal process.

（3）术野常规消毒，铺巾。

Disinfecting and draping in treatmental area as usual.

（4）针具：Ⅰ型 4 号针刀。

Acupotomy：Type Ⅰ-4 acupotomy.

（5）针刀操作。

Manipulation of acupotomy.

①腰椎小关节点：刀口线与人体纵轴一致，垂直进针。针刀经皮肤、皮下组织、肌肉达腰椎小关节关节囊骨面后，行"十"字切开，范围 0.5 cm。

Facet joint of lumbar vertebrae：Edge line direction of the acupotomy must be the same as the body axis. Practitioner inserts the acupotomy perpendicular to the bony surface of the lumbar facet joint capsule through skin，subcutaneous tissue and fascia nuchae to make a cross cut within 0.5 cm range.

②第三腰椎（L3）横突点：刀口线与人体纵轴一致，垂直进针，针刀尖落在横突骨面后，再向外移动针尖至横突尖部，向深部约 0.5 cm 处刺数下。

L3 transverse process：Edge line direction of the acupotomy must be the same as the body axis. Practitioner inserts the acupotomy perpendicular to the bony surface of the transverse process through skin, subcutaneous tissue and turns the needle tip outward to touch tip of the transverse process, and cuts several times within 0.5 cm in depth.

③第四至第五腰椎（L4～L5）和第五腰椎至第一骶骨（L5～S1）棘间韧带点：针刀体与皮肤垂直，先后从第五腰椎（L5）和第一骶骨（S1）棘突顶点进针刀，刀口线与脊柱纵轴平行，针刀经皮肤、皮下组织，直达棘突骨面，贴棘突上缘斜刺，深度约 0.5 cm；再向棘突下缘斜刺，深度约 0.5 cm；最后贴骨面向棘突两侧分别用提插刀法切割3 刀，深度 0.5 cm。

L4～L5 and L5～S1 ligamentas interspinalia: Edge line direction of the acupotomy must be the same as the body axis. Acupotomy is inserted perpendicular to the top of spinal process of L5 and S1 through skin, subcutaneous tissue. Practitioner turns the needle tip upward to superior side of the spinal process within 0.5 cm in depth, and then turns the needle tip downward to inferior side of the spinal process within 0.5 cm in depth, at last turns the needle tip to both side of the spinal process within 0.5 cm in depth to perform a three-cut with lifting-thrusting method.

注意：不能深刺至黄韧带，以免刺入椎管内。

Attention: Insertion of acupotomy must not be punched into the ligamentum flavum to avoid impingement of the spinal canal.

④竖脊肌起点：刀口线与人体纵轴一致，垂直进针，经皮肤、皮下组织到达竖脊肌，每个点上切割 3 刀。

Erector spinae: Edge line direction of the acupotomy must be the same as the body axis. Practitioner inserts the acupotomy perpendicular to the erector muscle of spine through skin, subcutaneous tissue, and then performs a three-cut on each point.

（6）针刀术后手法治疗。

Manipulation post-acupotomy treatment.

斜扳法，见第 41 页"急性腰椎后关节滑膜嵌顿"一节（图 2 - 24）。

Oblique pulling manipulation：Please refer to the chapter "Acute Lumbar Facet Joint Synovial"（Figure 2 - 24）.

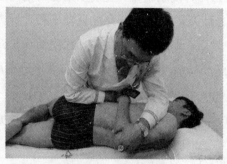

图 2 - 24 腰椎手法

Figure 2 - 24 Manual manipulation for lumbar vertebrae

9 腰椎滑脱症与峡部裂 Spondylolisthesis and Spondylolysis

【概述】Overview

腰椎滑脱症是指一个椎体在另一椎体上方向前滑脱。腰椎峡部裂以椎弓峡部断裂为特征，可导致腰椎滑脱。

Spondylolisthesisis is the slipping forward of one vertebra upon another. Spondylolysis is characterized by the presence of a bony defect at the pars interarticularis，which can result in spondylolisthesis.

9.1 峡部裂性腰椎滑脱症 Isthmic Spondylolisthesis

峡部裂性腰椎滑脱症的病因可能是发育性的，某些人群有峡部裂先天缺陷的发育不良易患因素。峡部裂在体操运动员、足球运动员、举重运动员和其他运动员中高发，由于他们的腰部常处于强力背伸状态，提示反复性的损伤是一个因素。生物力学研究也表明，在强力背伸状态下，关节间的峡部承受最大的压力。

The etiology of isthmic spondylolisthesis may be developmental, with a congenital defect of dysplasia predisposing on individuals to spondylolysis. The high incidence of spondylolysis in gymnasts, football players, weight lifters, and other athletes who post their lumbar spines in hyperextension suggests that repetitive injury may be a contributing mechanism. Biomechanical studies have also suggested that the pars interarticularis is under the greatest stress in extension.

【诊断要点】Keys to Diagnosis

腰椎滑脱症与腰椎峡部裂可能无临床症状，或可出现腰腿痛。极少情况下，出现根性症状，或肠道和膀胱症状。峡部裂性腰椎滑脱症最常发生在 10～15 岁青春发育期的迅速生长过程。滑脱程度与疼痛的严重程度不一定相关。第五腰椎（L5）峡部裂，即第五腰椎（L5）在骶椎上向前滑脱，最为常见。

Spondylolisthesis and spondylolysis may be asymptomatic, or they may present with back pain and leg pain. Rarely, they present with radicular symptoms or bowel and bladder symptoms. Isthmic spondylolisthesis presents most commonly during the preadolescent growth spurt, between the ages of 10 and 15. The extent of lippage may not be correlated with the severity of pain. The L5 pars interarticularis defect, with resultant slippage of L5 forward on the sacrum, is most commonly seen.

在年轻患者中，无论滑脱程度如何，可有腘绳肌紧张、屈膝、屈髋步态，即 Phalen-Dikson 征。仔细触诊腰椎滑脱症病人可发现其第五腰椎（L5）棘突上方有阶梯样错位。对于严重的滑脱症，腰骶部有明显的后凸、躯干变短、胸腔靠近髂嵴。

In young patients, regardless of the extent of slippage, there may be tight hamstrings and a knee-bent, hips-flexed gait, the classic Phalen-Dikson sign. Careful palpation of the spine of the patient with spondylolisthesis may reveal a step-off secondary to the prominent spinous process of L5. With more severe slippage, the lumbosacral junction becomes more kyphotic and the trunk appears shortened, with the rib cage approcaching the iliac crests.

放射检查侧位片将显示缺损，滑脱百分比测量也在此位，Meyerding's 分级法最常应用。斜位片将显示"项圈"或"断颈"的"斯柯特狗"。如果只是单侧缺损，对侧的峡部或椎板将显示硬化。如果有压缩骨折的病史但放射学检查阴性，骨扫描会有用。CT 影像上峡部裂呈一个不完整的环状。

Radiographic examination will show the defect on the lateral view, with the percentage of lippage measurable from this view. Meyerding's classification is the most commonly used. Oblique radiographs will demonstrate the "collar" or "broken neck" on the "Scottie dog". If a unilateral defect is present, the contralateral pars or lamina may show sclerosis. If the history is suggestive of an early stress fracture and radiographic findings are negative, bone scans may be useful. CT scanning will show spondylolysis as an incomplete ring.

麦氏分度法：

Ⅰ度滑脱：1%～25%；

Ⅱ度滑脱：26%～50%；

Ⅲ度滑脱：51%～75%；

Ⅳ度滑脱：76%～100%。

Meyerding's classification of degree of slippage in spondylolisthesis:

Grade Ⅰ is 1%～25% slippage;

Grade Ⅱ is 26%～50% slippage;

Grade Ⅲ is 51%～75% slippage;

Grade Ⅳ is 76%～100% slippage.

9.2 退变性腰椎滑脱症 Degenerative Spondylolisthesis

与峡部裂性腰椎滑脱症不同，退变性腰椎滑脱症多见于第四至第五腰椎（L4～L5）水平，由多种原因继发。这一水平比其他腰椎节段所受压力更大，因为第五腰椎至第一骶骨（L5～S1）水平有强大的翼状韧带保护，此韧带从第五腰椎（L5）横突起，止于髂骨翼；还因腰骶结合部低于髂嵴水平，在运动中得到保护。腰椎在上述水平上下的节段因活动结构多而分散了压力。在某种程度上，椎间盘和关节突关节发生退行性变的机率相对较高，椎间盘性狭窄会发生。由于关节突关节的结构和腰椎前凸，引发椎体向前滑移。

Unlike isthmic spondylolisthesis, degenerative spondylolisthesis is found more commonly at the L4～L5 level. This appears to be secondary to a number of factors. This level sees more stresses than other lumbar levels because the L5～S1 level is protected by the strong trasverse-alar ligaments that run from the transverse process of L5 to the sacral ala and also because the lumbosacral junction unually lies below the iliac crest and is additionally protected from motion. Other lumbar levels have more motion segments above and below to disperse stress. With degeneration at the disk and facet joints occurring at a somewhat greater rate, narrowing of the disk can occur. Because of the configuration of the facet joint and the lumbar lordosis, this results in some slippage forward of the vertebral body upon the one below.

椎间盘水平的狭窄可引起小关节压力增大，因而发生小关节退行性病变，包括小关节关节间隙狭窄和肥大、黄韧带肥厚赘生物，从而引起椎管狭窄。一个椎体在另一个椎体上方向前错位，进一步使椎管狭窄。

The narrowing at the disk level can lead to increased stresses at the facet joints, with resultant degenerative facet disease, including joint narrowing and hypertrophy of the facets and the redundant ligamentum flavum can result in spinal stenosis. The forward displacement of one vertebra upon the other can further narrow the canal.

大多数退行性滑脱患者表现出感觉减退或腿痛等椎管狭窄症候，椎管狭窄症的疼痛经常在步行一定距离后出现，坐下或弯腰时即能缓解。

Most patients with degenerative spondylolisthesis demonstrate an element of spinal stenosis symptomatology with dysesthesias or leg pian. The spinal stenosis pattern of pain when walking beyond a well-defined distance (neurogenic claudication) is often present and relieved only by sitting down or bending over.

【小针刀治疗】Acupotomy therapy

适用于Ⅰ～Ⅱ度的腰椎前滑脱患者，其他患者则需手术治疗。

Acupotomy therapy is suitable for spondylolisthesis with grade Ⅰ to Ⅱ. Of course, surgery may be indicated for other severe cases.

操作方法：

Procedure：

（1）体位：俯卧位（图 2 - 25）。

Posture：Prone position（Figure 2 - 25）.

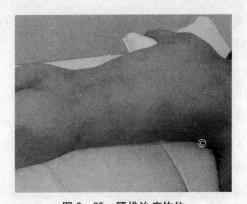

图 2 – 25　腰椎治疗体位

Figure 2 – 25　Posture for lumbal vertebrae

（2）定位（图 2 – 26）。

Location（Figure 2 – 26）.

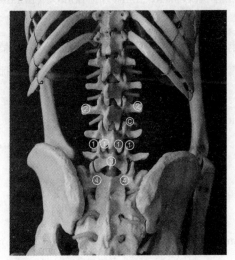

图 2 – 26　腰椎滑脱症与峡部裂进针定点

Figure 2 – 26　Inserting points for spondylolisthesis & spondylolysis

①腰椎小关节　Facet joint of lumbar vertebrae；②L3 横突点　L3 transverse process；③L4～L5、L5～S1 棘间韧带点　　L4～L5 and L5～S1 ligamentas interspinalia；④竖脊肌起点　Erector spinae

①腰椎小关节：第四腰椎（L4）棘突和第五腰椎（L5）棘突最高点水平，正中线旁分别开1 cm、2 cm，即小关节内侧、外侧，两侧各取 2 点。

Facet joint of lumbar vertebrae：On the top of spinal processes of L4 and L5，mark two points 1 cm lateral and 2 cm lateral the midline on each side. Those points autruely locate at interior side and exterior side of the facet joint.

②第三腰椎（L3）、第四腰椎（L4）和第五腰椎（L5）横突点：分别在第二至第三腰椎（L2～L3）、第三至第四腰椎（L3～L4）和第四至第五腰椎（L4～L5）棘间隙，正中线旁开 3 cm，两侧各取 1 点。

L3，L4 and L5 transverse processes：Between L2～L3，L3～L4 and L4～L5 spinal processes，mark one point 3 cm lateral the midline on each side.

③第四至第五腰椎（L4～L5）、第五腰椎至第一骶骨（L5～S1）棘间韧带点：第五腰椎（L5）和第一骶骨（S1）棘突顶点，后正中线上。

L4～L5 and L5～S1 ligamentas interspinalia：Two points on the top of L5 and S1 spinal process in the midline posteriorly will be chosen.

④竖脊肌起点：第五腰椎（L5）棘突下方骶中嵴，中线旁开 2cm 各取 1 点。

Erector spinae：Mark two points 2 cm lateral the midline on each side，at cristae sacralis media level which locates below the L5 spinal process.

（3）术野常规消毒，铺巾。

Disinfecting and draping in treatmental area as usual.

（4）针具：Ⅰ型 4 号针刀。

Acupotomy：Type Ⅰ-4 acupotomy.

（5）针刀操作。

Manipulation of acupotomy.

①腰椎小关节点：刀口线与人体纵轴一致，垂直进针。针刀经皮肤、皮下组织、肌肉达腰椎小关节关节囊骨面后，沿脊柱纵轴方向切3刀，范围0.5 cm。

Facet joint of lumbar vertebrae: Edge line direction of the acupotomy must be the same as the body axis. Practitioner inserts the acupotomy perpendicular to the bony surface of the lumbar facet joint capsule through skin, subcutaneous tissue and fascia nuchae to perform a three-cut along the spinal axis within 0.5 cm.

②第三腰椎（L3）、第四腰椎（L4）和第五腰椎（L5）横突点：刀口线与人体纵轴一致，垂直进针，针刀尖落在横突骨面后，再向外移动针尖至横突尖部，向深部0.5 cm刺数下。

L3, L4 and L5 transverse processes: Edge line direction of the acupotomy must be the same as the body axis. Practitioner inserts the acupotomy perpendicular to the bony surface of the transverse process through skin, subcutaneous tissue and turns the needle tip outward to touch tip of the transverse process, and cuts several times within 0.5 cm in depth.

③第四至第五腰椎（L4～L5）和第五腰椎至第一骶骨（L5～S1）棘间韧带点：针刀体与皮肤垂直，先后从第五腰椎（L5）和第一骶骨（S1）棘突顶点进针刀，刀口线与脊柱纵轴平行，针刀经皮肤、皮下组织，直达棘突骨面，贴棘突上缘斜刺，深度约0.5 cm；再向棘突下缘斜刺，深度约0.5 cm；最后贴骨面向棘突两侧分别用提插刀法切割3刀，深度约0.5 cm。

L4～L5 and L5～S1 ligamentas interspinalia: Edge line direction of the acupotomy must be the same as the body axis. Acupotomy is inserted perpendicular to the top of spinal process of L5 and S1 through skin, subcutaneous tissue. Practitioner turns the needle tip upward to superior side of the spinal process within 0.5 cm in depth, and then turns the needle tip downward to inferior side of the spinal process within 0.5 cm in depth, at last turns the needle tip to both side of the spinal process within 0.5 cm in depth to perform a three-cut with lift-cutting method.

注意：不能深刺至黄韧带，以免刺入椎管内。

Attention: Insertion of acupotomy must not be punched into the ligamentum flavum to avoid impingement of the spinal canal.

④竖脊肌起点：刀口线与人体纵轴一致，垂直进针，经皮肤、皮下组织到达竖脊肌，每个点上切割 3 刀。

Erector spinae: Edge line direction of the acupotomy must be the same as the body axis. Practitioner inserts the acupotomy perpendicular to the erector muscle of spine through skin, subcutaneous tissue, and then performs a three-cut on each point.

（6）针刀术后手法治疗。

Manipulation post-acupotomy treatment.

仰卧位冲压法：适用于第四腰椎（L4）、第五腰椎（L5） Ⅰ～Ⅱ度的退变性前滑脱（无椎弓峡部裂）患者。患者仰卧，双手叠放于腹部，腰骶部垫一薄枕，屈髋屈膝。术者嘱患者吸气后屏住，用手压在患者双膝处，向下冲压患者腹部 3 次（图 2-27）。

Push and pressure in a prone position: This manipulation is suitable for degenerative spondylolisthesis with grade Ⅰ to Ⅱ in L4 or L5 level (There is not bony defect at the pars interarticularis). Patient lying in a supine position with a thin pillow under his waist, and crossing both arms on his stomach and flexing both hips and knees above, a practitioner presses patient's knees with one hand, asks patient breathing-in and holding, and then performs downward push and pressure for 3 times （Figure 2 - 27）.

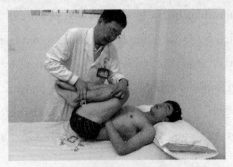

图 2 - 27　腰椎滑脱症仰卧位冲压法

Figure 2 - 27　Manipulation of push and pressure in a prone position

10　冈上肌肌腱炎　Tendinitis of Supraspinatus Muscle

【概述】Overview

冈上肌肌腱炎是由于肩部运动不当，冈上肌腱受肩峰摩擦，导致肌腱和肩峰下滑囊损伤并发炎，引起患者肩部外展时出现疼痛的病症。

Tendinitis of supraspinatus muscle results in friction between supraspinatus muscle acromion because of improper movement of shoulder. Injury of the tendon and the subacromial bursa result in irritation and inflammation, and which lead to patient showing a painful disorder while shoulder abduction.

冈上肌活动于上肢各种形式的提升。肩关节外展时，肩峰下滑囊回缩到近端，使冈上肌腱直接与肩峰骨面接触，并在肩峰下面和肱骨头上面的狭小间隙内受到肩峰和喙肩韧带的摩擦，病人产生肩部外侧疼痛；肩外展时疼痛明显等症状。

75

The supraspinatus muscle is active in all patterns of arm elevation. Subacromial bursa is withdrowed proximal during shoulder abduction, which leads to tendinitis of supraspinatus muscle meeting acromion directly, and the tendonitis is abraded by acromion and acromiocoracoid ligament in a narrow space beneath acromion and above caput humeri. Patient complaints painful shoulder in lateral side and the pain getting worse obviously during shoulder abduction.

【诊断要点】Keys to diagnosis

（1）上臂外侧疼痛，外展 60°～120°时明显。

The patient complains painful lateral side of the upper arm and pain getting obvious when shoulder abducting in range 60 to 120 degrees.

（2）患侧肩峰外下方有明显压痛，肩关节主动活动可受限，但被动活动不受限。

Pressure pain can be found at acromion process of affected side obviously. Active motion of shoulder joint is limited but the passivity one is fine.

（3）有的病例在 X 射线片上可见到肱骨大结节处有钙化影。

On X-ray film a calcify shadow can be seen near great tuberosity in some cases.

【小针刀治疗】Acupotomy therapy

（1）体位：侧卧位（图 2 - 28）。

Posture：Lateral position (Figure 2 - 28).

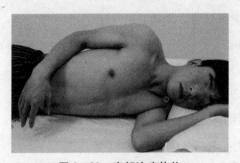

图 2 - 28 肩部治疗体位

Figure 2 - 28 Posture for shoulder

（2）定点。

Location.

肩峰下压痛点：肩峰下缘压痛最明显处（图 2 - 29）。

The point can be found in the most obvious tender area inferior border in acromion (Figure 2 - 29).

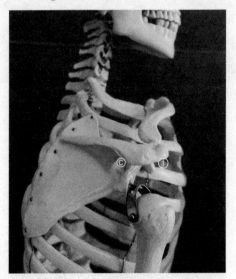

图 2 - 29 冈上肌腱炎进针定点

Figure 2 - 29 Inserting points for tendinitis of supraspinatus muscle

①肩峰下压痛点 Tender point inferior border in acromion

（3）术野常规消毒，铺巾。

Disinfecting and draping in treatmental area as usual.

（4）针具：Ⅰ型4号针刀。

Acupotomy：Type Ⅰ-4 acupotomy.

（5）针刀操作。

Manipulation of acupotomy.

肩峰下压痛点：针刀与皮面垂直，刀口线肌纤维方向一致，贴肩峰下缘骨面刺入，深度1 cm，纵向分离肌腱周围粘连。

Tender area in acromion：The acupotomy being vertical to the skin surface，with the cutting line being in concord with the direction of the muscle fiber，then closely insert the blade with inferior border of acromion in 1 cm depth，for dissection of nearby adhered tendon.

（6）术后手法。

Manipulation post-acupotomy treatment.

施术者立于患侧，一手持患肘，作对抗牵引外展，并做肩部旋前旋后活动（图2-30）。

Standing on affected side，performer holds patient's elbow to countertract and moves patient's shoulder abducted，pronated and supinated（Figure 2-30）.

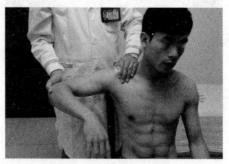

图2-30　肩部手法

Figure 2-30　Manual manipulation for shoulder

11　肩关节周围炎　Periarthritis of Shoulder

【概述】Overview

肩关节周围炎又称"冻结肩"，常见于老年人，尤其是 50 岁左右的女性。病人表现为肩关节疼痛和逐渐加重的肩关节活动受限。

Periarthritis of shoulder is also called Frozen Shoulder and is most frequently seen in the older people，especially women in their fifth decades. Patients suffer painful shoulder and progressive limitation in the range of motion of the shoulder joint.

肩关节周围炎始于肩部的任何原因导致的炎症过程，其临床本质是肩关节囊的粘连。这种原发于关节囊的炎症使肩关节活动逐渐受限。此病一般经历关节囊疤痕期、关节纤维化期和修复期 3 个病理过程，过程可达 18～24 个月。

For periarthritis of shoulder，adhesive capsulitis is a clinical entity that begins with any type of inflammatory process about the shoulder. The inflammation leads to progressive limitation in the range of motion of the shoulder joint，primarily in the capsule. The disease is classically described as three phases：capsular scar，fibrous arthrodesis，recovery. The process is 18～24 months.

【诊断要点】Keys to diagnosis

（1）肩部疼痛，夜间尤甚，且多发于中老年人。

Sore shoulder，especially at night，which attacks middle-aged and senile people.

（2）肩关节活动受限或僵硬，尤以肩外展、上举、外旋明显。

Motive range of shoulder is limited or stiff that is obvious in abduction，lift and extorsion.

（3）如病程较长者，可见肩胛带肌萎缩，尤以三角肌萎缩明显。

Muscles of shoulder girdle，especially in deltoid，are atrophied if course of diseases last long.

【小针刀治疗】Acupotomy therapy

（1）体位：端坐位（图2-31）。

Posture：Sit straight （Figure 2-31）.

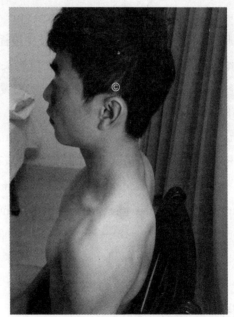

图2-31　肩部治疗体位

Figure 2-31　Posture for shoulder

（2）定点。

Location.

①喙突：喙突顶点，其外下方肱二头肌短头起点有明显压痛。

Coracoid process：The point can be found in the outer lower area of its peak，near starting point of biceps brachii short head with the most obvious tender.

②肱骨小结节：喙突向外触及的第一个骨突即是肱骨小结节。

Lesser tubercle humerus：in the first follicle of the reach point of coracoid process.

③结节间沟：位于肱骨大结节、小结节之间，通常有明显压痛。

Intertubercular sulcus：In space between greater and lesser tubercle，with the most obvious tender.

④肱骨大结节小圆肌止点：喙突向外触及的第二个骨突即是肱骨大结节。小圆肌止点位于肱骨大结节后下方。

End point of teres minor in greater tubercle：The greater tubercle is located in the second follicle of the reach point of coracoid process，and the end point of teres minor is located in the lower rear of the former.

⑤肩胛骨：冈上肌、冈下肌和小圆肌部位的压痛点。

Shoulder blade：Tenderness points in muscles may be located in the supraspinatus，infraspinatus and teres minor.

将选定的治疗点用记号笔标明（图 2 - 32）。

Mark all selected points with a marker (Figure 2 - 32).

（3）术野常规消毒，铺巾。

Disinfecting and draping in treatmental area as usual.

（4）针具：Ⅰ型 4 号针刀。

Acupotomy：Type Ⅰ -4 acupotomy.

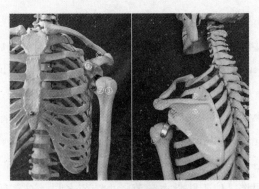

图 2 - 32　肩部进针定点

Figure 2 - 32　Inserting points for shoulder

①喙突　Coracoid process；②肱骨小结节　Lesser tubercle humerus；③结节间沟　Intertubercular sulcus；④肱骨大结节小圆肌止点　End point of teres minor in greater tubercle；⑤肩胛骨　Shoulder blade

（5）针刀操作。

Manipulation of acupotomy.

①喙突：喙突顶点进针，针体与皮肤垂直，刀口线与上肢纵轴平行。刺至喙突顶点骨面后，针尖贴其外侧 1/3 肱二头肌短头起点刺入，纵疏横剥 3 刀，范围 0.5cm。

Coracoid process：Insert the needle vertically with the skin surface in its peak，with the cutting line being parallel with longitudinal axis of the upper limb. Stop until reaching the bony surface，then move the needle point to 1/3 of biceps brachii short head，make a three-cut for dredging lengthwise and seperating broadwise in around 0.5 cm.

②肱骨小结节：在缘突外侧，针刀在触及肱骨小结节肩胛下肌止点刺入，直达肱骨小结节骨面，纵疏横剥 3 刀，范围 0.5 cm。

Lesser tubercle humerus：outside the coracoid process，insert the needle blade in the point touching end point of lower shoulder blade muscle in lesser tubercle humerus，continue until reaching bony surface of the lesser tubercle humerus, then make a three-cut for dredging lengthwise and seperating broadwise in 0.5 cm range around.

③结节间沟：肱骨大结节、小结节之间，可触及肱二头肌长头肌腱。针刀体与皮肤垂直，刀口线与上肢纵轴一致，直达肱骨结节间沟前面的骨面，先用提插刀法松解 3 刀。

Intertubercular sulcus: between greater and lesser tubercle, in the space possible to touch biceps brachii long head tendon, cutting line with the longitudinal axis of the upper limb, continue until reaching intertubercular sulcus of the humerus, followed by 3 lifting-thrusting cuts for relief.

④小圆肌止点：肱骨大结节后下方进针，针刀体与皮肤垂直，刀口线与上肢纵轴一致，刺达肱骨大结节后下方的小圆肌止点，用提插刀法松解 3 刀。

End point of teres in greater tubercle: Insert an acupotomy to the lower rear part of the greater tubercle, needle boby being perpendicular to the skin and needle blade being the same as limb axis. When inserting to the ending of teres in lower rear part of the greater tubercle, make a three-cut with lifting-thrusting method.

⑤肩胛骨：顺着冈上肌、冈下肌和小圆肌肌纤维方向，垂直刺入针刀至上述肌肉痛点，每个点刺 3 下，范围约 0.5 cm。

Shoulder blade: Along the fiber direction of the supraspinatus, infraspinatus and teres minor, insert acupotomy vertically to those tenderness points and make a three-cut in 0.5 cm range in each point.

术毕，拔出针刀，局部压迫止血 3 分钟后，用创可贴覆盖针眼。

When acupotomy treatment has finished, practitioner withdraws the acupotomy and applies pressure to the treated points for three minutes and adhesive dressing such as a Band-Aid.

注意：

①喙突处松解喙突顶点范围只有 0.8 cm 左右，但却有 5 个肌肉、

韧带的起止点，针刀对肩周炎的喙突松解部位位于喙突的外 1/3 处，以松解到肱二头肌短头起点。如果在中 1/3 处或者内 1/3 处松解，则难以起效，还可能损伤其他组织。

Attentions：

The theraputic area of dissection in coracoid process peak is only about 0. 8 cm，however，there are 5 muscles covered and the start point and end point of the ligaments around；in addition，the dissection point in coracoid process peak for acupotomy therapy is started in the outer 1/3 of the peak，and ended in biceps brachii short head. Thus，if the start point moved to middle or inner part，the therapy would not take effect，even do harm to other tissues.

②防止头静脉损伤。头静脉起于手背静脉网的桡侧，沿前臂桡侧上行至肘窝，在肱二头肌外侧沟内继续上行，经过三角肌胸大肌间沟，再穿锁胸筋膜汇入腋静脉或者锁骨下静脉。在做肱骨小结节处肩胛下肌止点松解及肱骨结节间沟处肱二头肌长头起点松解时，表面是头静脉的走行路线。预防头静脉损伤的方法是先摸清楚三角肌胸大肌间沟，旁开 0. 5 cm 进针刀，严格按照四步操作规程进针刀，即可避免损伤头静脉。

Prevent possible cephalic vein injury. Cephalic vein starts in radialis of the back hand vein net，moving upward through forearm radialis to axillary fossa，and continues to rise inside the lateral groove of the biceps brachii，then passes intergroove between deltoid muscle and pectoralis major，finally merged with axillary vein or subclavian vein throught clavipectoral fascia. When dissecting end point of lower shoulder blade muscle in lesser tubercle humerus and start point of biceps brachii long head in biceps groove，the surface for cutting is the route of cephalic vein. To prevent possible injury，the operator should clearly locate intergroove between deltoid muscle and pectoralis major，then insert the needle blade at 0. 5 cm distance， following the Four Steps for Acupotomy Manipulation strictly，which could probably avoid such injury.

（6）针刀术后手法治疗。

Manipulation post-acupotomy treatment.

施术者一只手扶住患者肩部，另一只手握患手，作牵引、抖动、旋转等活动，并帮助患肢做外展、外旋、上举、前屈、后伸等动作（图 2 - 33）。

Performer fixes patient's shoulder with one hand and grasps affected hand with the other hand to tractate，shake and rotate. Then helps patient to abduct，extort，lift，flex and extend the shoulder （Figure 2 - 33）.

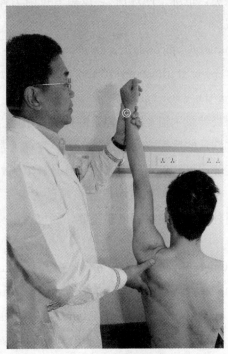

图 2 - 33　肩部手法

Figure 2 - 33　Manual manipulation for shoulder

注意：协助患肢作活动时要循序渐进，以免引起局部组织再次损伤而发生进一步粘连。

Attention：Helping affected arm to move in proper sequence in order to avoid being adhesion due to local tissue injury again.

12 肱骨外上髁炎（网球肘） External Humeral Epicondylitis（Tennis Elbow）

【概述】Overview

肱骨外上髁炎，也称"网球肘"，以患者抗阻力伸腕时肱骨外上髁处疼痛为特点。

External humeral epicondylitis is also known as Tennis Elbow characterized by pain at the lateral humeral epicondyle produced by patient extending the wrist against resistance.

肱骨外上髁炎涉及手指及腕部伸肌的伸肌总肌腱。患者频繁抗阻力背伸腕部（如网球的反手击球）最易引发。疼痛通常实质上是慢性的，而且比功能障碍更恼人，压痛点位于肱骨外上髁处，疼痛由抗阻力伸腕而引发。桡侧腕短伸肌肌腱已经被确认为最常见的病损部位。其他一些引起肘外侧疼痛的病因也要查明，如桡骨小头关节炎和骨间后神经卡压。

External humeral epicondylitis involves the common tendon to the extensor muscles of the wrist and hand. Patients who perform repetitive wrist extension against resistance (such as the backhand stroke in tennis) are at risk. The pain they have is usually chronic in nature and more bothersome than disabling. Tenderness is located over the lateral humeral epicondyle and pain produced by extending the wrist against resistance. The tendon of the extensor carpi radialis brevis has been identified as the most common site of the lesion. Other causes for lateral elbow pain should be looked for, including radiocapitellar arthritis and posterior interosseous nerve compression.

【诊断要点】 Keys to diagnosis

(1) 患肘外侧肱骨外上髁局部持续性酸痛。

The patient complains of continuous ache at epicondylus extensorius of affected elbow.

(2) 局部压痛，前臂抗阻力的伸直和旋转可使疼痛加重。

Pressure pain is found at local part and pains getting worse by forearm are antagonistic extending or rotating.

【小针刀治疗】 Acupotomy therapy

(1) 体位：卧位，将肘关节屈曲 90°平放于治疗桌面上（图 2 - 34）。

Posture：Patient lies in bed, with his elbow leaning on the table and flexing 90 degrees (Figure 2 - 34).

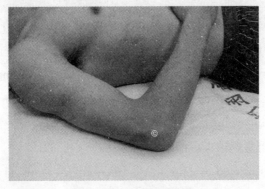

图 2 - 34　肘部治疗体位

Figure 2 - 34　Posture for elbow

（2）定点（图 2 - 35）。

Location（Figure 2 - 35）.

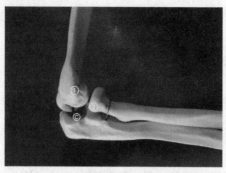

图 2 - 35　肱骨外上髁进针定点

Figure 2 - 35　Inserting points for epicondylus extensorius

①肱骨外上髁顶点　The lateral epicondyle of humerus vertex；②肱骨外上髁远端痛点　The lateral epicondyle of humerus distal pain points

①肱骨外上髁顶点定 1 点。

Mark one point in the lateral epicondyle of humerus vertex.

②肱骨外上髁远端痛点：嘱患者抗阻力做伸指伸腕动作，沿肱骨外上髁远端 2 cm 范围内，在腕、指伸肌腱起点找出 1～2 个痛点作为进针点。

The lateral epicondyle of humerus distal pain points：Asking the patient to stretch his fingers and wrist with the force resisting the drag，one or two points are marked in the wrist and finger extensor tendon point 2 cm away from the lateral epicondyle of humerus distal as the inserting point.

（3）术野常规消毒，铺巾。

Disinfecting and draping in treatmental area as usual.

（4）针具：Ⅰ型 4 号针刀。

Acupotomy：Type Ⅰ-4 acupotomy.

（5）针刀操作。

Manipulation of acupotomy.

肱骨外上髁顶点：针刀刀口线和前臂纵轴方向一致，针刀垂直刺至肱骨外上髁顶点，纵行提插切割 3 刀。

The lateral epicondyle of humerus vertex：Cutting line being consistent with forearm longitudinal axis. Then insert the blade vertically into the lateral epicondyle of humerus vertex，followed by a three-cut lifting and thrusting cuts along longitudinal axis.

肱骨外上髁远端痛点：在肱骨外上髁远端压痛明显处，刀口线和前臂纵轴方向一致，针刀垂直经皮肤、皮下组织，达腕、指伸肌肌间隙，纵行提插切割 3 刀，范围 0.5 cm。

The lateral epicondyle of humerus distal pain points：In part of the lateral epicondyle of humerus distal with obvious tenderness，make the cutting line consistent with forearm longitudinal axis，then insert the blade vertically through skin and subcutaneous tissue until reaching gap between wrist and finger extensor muscle，followed by three lifting and thrusting cuts in the longitudinal axis within the range of 0.5 cm.

术毕，拔出针刀，局部压迫止血 3 分钟后，用创可贴覆盖针眼。

When acupotomy treatment is finished，practitioner withdraws the acupotomy and applies pressure to the treated points for three minutes and adhesive dressing such as a Band-Aid.

注意：肱骨外上髁炎 3 次针刀治疗可痊愈，若 3 次针刀治疗后无明显疗效，就应考虑是否合并颈椎病，再仔细询问病史，检查患侧上肢有无感觉过敏或感觉迟钝，如有颈椎病等其他临床表现，应按颈椎病进行针刀治疗。

Attention：Humeral epicondylitis can be cured by 3 times of acupotomy treatment normally. If the symptom continue to exist with no obvious improvement after 3 times of treatment, complication of cervical spondylosis should be considered, which is suggested to re-examine the patient's the medical history for any possible senseless or slowness in the upper limb. If clinical manifestation of cervical spondylosis diagnosed, acupotomy treatment in cervical spondylosis should be carried out.

（6）针刀术后手法治疗。

Manipulation post-acupotomy treatment.

使前臂旋前、旋后动作数次（图 2 - 36）。

Pronating and supinating his/her forearm several times (Figure 2 - 36).

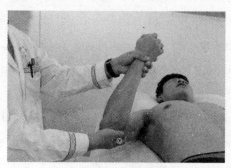

图 2 - 36　肘部手法

Figure 2 - 36　Manual manipulation for elbow

注意：手法宜由轻到重，轻揉缓和，切忌粗暴手法。

Attention：Strength of manipulation should be played from light to hard, gentle but not wild.

13　桡骨茎突腱鞘炎　Tenosynovitis of Styloid Process of Radius

【概述】 Overview

　　桡骨茎突部为外展拇长肌肌腱与拇短伸肌肌腱腱鞘通过。由于腕部活动,上述两肌腱在其共同腱鞘中频繁活动而致劳损,使局部充血、肿胀、发炎,影响肌腱活动而出现桡骨茎突部疼痛,活动不便。

The abductor pollicis longus and extensor pollicis brevis tendons share the same epitenon at the radial styloid region. Two tendons mention above will get congestion, edema and inflammation by strain resulting from wrist overuse. Painful wrist at local region and limitated movement of wrist are produced by lesions of those involved tendons and epitenon.

　　由于拇长展肌腱和拇短伸肌腱在桡骨茎突部的伸肌支持带下发炎,在腕部尺偏、拇指内收和屈曲时的提升动作将会引发桡骨茎突部疼痛。做一些活动时,如排空血压计袖带、从婴儿床抱起新生儿或从烤箱中取出沉重的托盘等动作,都会引发腕部桡侧的疼痛。

The abductor pollicis longus and extensor pollicis brevis tendons may become inflamed beneath the retinacular pulley at the radial styloid region. Pain at the radial styloid is provoked by lifting activity in which the thumb is adducted and flexed while the hand is ulnarly deviated. Activities such as inflating a blood pressue cuff, picking up a new baby out of a crib, or lifting a heavy frying pan off the stove may provoke pain along the radial aspect of the wrist.

【诊断要点】Keys to diagnosis

（1）腕部用力提物时疼痛。

Painful wrist is produced while lifting a heavy matter.

（2）桡骨茎突处压痛，可摸到硬结节。

Tenderness and induration are found at the radial styloid area.

（3）芬克斯坦（Finkelstein）试验对诊断此病有帮助。

The Finkelstein test may be helpful in diagnosing this disorder.

【小针刀治疗】Acupotomy therapy

（1）体位：仰卧位，患者握拳，将患侧腕部放于治疗桌面上（图 2 - 37）。

Posture：Dorsal position，patient's affected side wrist was put on the table while clenching his fist（Figure 2 - 37）.

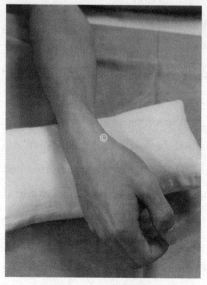

图 2 - 37　腕部治疗体位

Figure 2 - 37　Posture for wrist

（2）定位：桡骨茎突压痛明显处（图 2－38）。

Location：The obvious painful point on radial styloid（Figure 2－38）.

（3）术野常规消毒，铺巾。

Disinfecting and draping in treatmental area as usual.

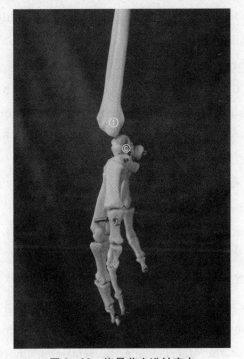

图 2－38　桡骨茎突进针定点

Figure 2－38　Inserting points for the radial styloid

①桡骨茎突　radial styloid

（4）针具：Ⅰ型 4 号针刀。

Acupotomy：Type Ⅰ-4 acupotomy.

（5）针刀操作。

Manipulation of acupotomy.

针刀刀口线与腕部纵轴平行，针刀垂直刺入桡骨茎突最高处，到达骨面后稍提起针尖，向远端用提插刀法在纤维鞘管上纵切数刀，感觉刀下有韧性感，范围约 1 cm。手术完毕，拔出针刀，局部压迫止血 3 分钟后，用创可贴覆盖针眼。

Cutting line is paralleled with the longitudinal axis of wrist, then piercing is vertical on the highest point of radial styloid. When reaching the bone surface, the acupotomy should be lifted up slightly and cuted longitudinally several times on the distal fibrous sheath by lifting and thrusting methods. Toughness will be sensed when cutting, and the cutting range is about 1 cm. When acupotomy treatment finished, practitioner withdraws the acupotomy and applies pressure to the treated points for three minutes and adhesive dressing such as a Band-Aid.

（6）针刀术后手法治疗。

Manipulation post-acupotomy treatment.

术后，施术者一只手握住患侧腕部，另一只手食指及中指夹持拇指，其余手指紧握患者其他四指进行对抗牵引，并使患者腕部向尺侧和掌侧屈曲，重复 3 次（图 2 - 39）。

After the acupotomy therapy, hold the affected wrist by one hand. And clamping the thumb of the patient by the index finger and middle finger of the other, while the remaining fingers are used to hold the patient's other four fingers to perform traction, along with flexing the patient's wrist to the ulnar and palmar. Repeat the above process 3 times (Figure 2 - 39).

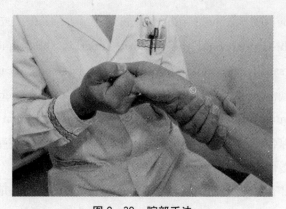

图 2 - 39 腕部手法

Figure 2 - 39 Manual manipulation for wrist

14 腕管综合征 Carpal Tunnel Syndrome

【概述】 Overview

腕管综合征是一种由于正中神经在腕管中受到卡压，引起的以拇指、食指和中指麻木，活动不利为主要症状的病症。

Carpal tunnel syndrome is a compression of the median nerve within the carpal tunnel，and which producing numbness and clumsiness in the thumb，index and middle fingers.

正中神经在腕管中受压是上肢最常见的神经压迫损伤。腕管的空间沿腕部掌侧行走，其解剖四边包括桡侧的舟骨结节、大多角骨，尺侧的豆状骨、钩骨钩突，背侧的月骨、三角骨以及掌侧的腕横韧带。腕管中有指浅屈肌、正中神经、拇长屈肌和指深屈肌通过。

Compression of the median nerve within the carpal tunnel is the most common upper extremity compressive neuropathy. The carpal tunnel is that space along the palmar aspect of the wrist anatomoically bounded by the scaphoid tubercle and the trapezium radially, the hook of the hamate and the pisiform ulnarly, the triquetrum and lunate dorsally, and the transverse carpal ligament on the palmar side. There are flexor digitorum superficialis, median nerve, flexor pollcis longus and flexor digitorum profundus within the carpal tunnel.

腕管综合征常呈突发，与妊娠、淀粉样病变、屈肌腱鞘炎、腕部劳损、急慢性炎症、损伤或腕管内的肿瘤有关。

Carpal tunnel syndrome is often idiopathic. It has been associated with pregnancy, amyloidosis, flexor tenosynovitis, overuse phenomenon, acute or chronic inflammatory conditions, traumatic disorders of the wrist, and tumors within the carpal tunnel.

【诊断要点】Keys to diagnosis

（1）腕部和拇指、食指、中指麻木、疼痛、肿胀，手部无力。

Numbed, painful and swollen sensation at wrist, thumb, point finger and middle finger, hand weakness.

（2）手部正中神经支配区的皮肤感觉减弱或消失。叩击腕部正中神经区呈放射性触电样刺痛及 Tinel's 征呈阳性，腕屈试验呈阳性。

Anaesthesia in dermatome of eneurosis of medianus nerve. Knocking patient's wrist would conduct stabbing pain like electric shock around eneurosis of medianus nerve. Tinel's sign and wrist flexing test are positive.

（3）X 射线检查可见有的病人可能有陈旧性桡骨远端骨折、月骨脱位或腕骨关节炎等。

X-ray signs: Some patients probably suffered from old radial fracture at distant end of the bone, old lunar bone dislocation or osteoarthritis of the wrist.

【小针刀治疗】 Acupotomy therapy

（1）体位：仰卧位，手掌向上，腕关节置于脉枕上（图 2 - 40）。

Position：Supinate，with palms and wrist on the pillow（Figure 2 - 40）.

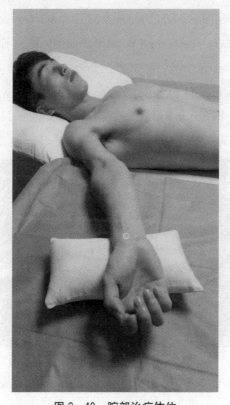

图 2 - 40　腕部治疗体位

Figure 2 - 40　Posture for wrist

（2）定位：让患者用力握拳屈腕，在腕部掌侧可有 3 条行皮下的隆起，中间为掌长肌腱，桡侧为桡侧腕屈肌腱，尺侧为尺侧腕屈肌腱。在远侧腕横纹尺侧腕屈肌腱的内侧缘，定下第一点，沿尺侧腕屈肌的内缘向远端移 2.5 cm 左右再定第二点；在远腕横纹上的桡侧腕屈肌腱的内侧缘定第三点，再沿桡侧腕屈肌腱向远端移动 2.5 cm 左右，定为第四点。此 4 点即为进针点（图 2 - 41）。

Location: Patient's fist being clenched while the wrist flexed, until 3 subcutaneous uplift observed in palmaris; divided by which, practitioner can distinguish palmaris longus tendon in the middle, radialis and ulnaris flex tendon in their corresponding sides. The first point is located in the medial margin of the distal wrist crease tendon of flex carpi ulnar, the second point is located along the inner edge of flex carpi ulnar muscle to the distal shift of about 2.5 cm; and the third point is in medial carpi in the far stripes of the wrist flex tendon edge, following by the fourth point is in 2.5 cm along the flex carpi radial tendon. Those four points are used for inserting (Figure 2 - 41).

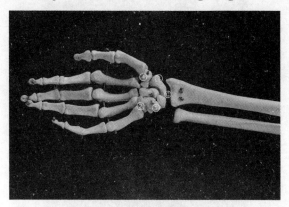

图 2 - 41 腕管综合征进针定点

Figure 2 - 41 Inserting points for Carpal Tunnel Syndrome

①~④腕部进针点 Inserting points for wrist

（3）术野常规消毒，铺巾。

Disinfecting and draping in treatmental area as usual.

（4）针具：Ⅰ型 4 号针刀。

Acupotomy: Type Ⅰ-4 acupotomy.

（5）针刀操作。

Manipulation of acupotomy.

在上述 4 点上分别进针刀，刀口线和肌腱走向平行，针体和腕平面成 90°，沿两侧屈肌内侧缘刺入 0.5 cm 左右，应避开尺动静脉、桡动静脉和神经，将腕横韧带分别切开 2～3 cm。

Needles are simultaneously inserted in the four points mentioned above, with the cutting edge line being parallel to the tendon, and the needle body being vertical to the wrist plane, then insert the needle along both sides of the medial margin for about 0.5 cm, beware to avoid the ulnar radial artery, vein and nerve, cutting is finished when the transverse carpal ligament is open 2～3 cm.

术毕压迫针眼 3 分钟，用创可贴覆盖创口。

When acupotomy treatment finished, practitioner applies pressure to the treated points for three minutes and adhesive dressing such as a Band-Aid.

（6）针刀术后手法治疗。

Manipulation post-acupotomy treatment.

施术者双手握患者掌部，右手在桡侧、左手在尺侧，而拇指平放于腕关节的背侧，以拇指指端按于关节背侧。在拔伸情况下摇晃关节。然后，将手在拇指按压下背伸至最大宽度，随即屈曲，并左、右各转 2～3 次（图 2 - 42）。

The palm of the patient is hold by the operator with his both hands, using right hand on the radial side, and the left hand on the ulnar side. In the meantime, the operator presses his/her dorsal joints with thumb, and then shakes them while pulling. Finally, use the thumb to press and to stretch the hand dorsal extension to the maximum width, followed by immediate bending, and turns around for 2～3 times (Figure 2 - 42).

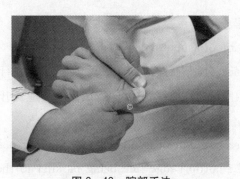

图 2 - 42　腕部手法

Figure 2 - 42　Manual manipulation for wrist

15　屈指肌腱腱鞘炎　Flexor Tenosynovitis（Trigger Finger）

【概述】Overview

屈指肌腱腱鞘炎俗称"弹响指""扳机指"，以掌侧近端屈肌腱鞘滑车部位疼痛和压痛为特征。患者常诉患指或拇指在强行屈指时被卡住并发生弹响。

Often called Stuck-Finger or Trigger Finger，flexor tenosynovitis is characterized by pain and tenderness in the palm at the proximal edge of the pulley. Patients frequently note catching or triggering of the affected finger or thumb after forceful flexion.

屈指肌腱腱鞘炎可发生于任一个屈指肌腱，在肌腱行走全程，更多在其骨纤维滑车部约束点，或在屈肌腱支持带鞘内，由手指屈曲活动频繁的刺激和炎症引起腱鞘狭窄所致。狭窄性腱鞘炎特别多见于糖尿病患者，当多个手指受累时，对于先前未确诊的患者必须考虑有患糖尿病的可能。

Flexor tenosynovitis may develop about any of the extrinsic flexor tendons, either throughout their course or, more commonly, at points of constraint by bony fibrous pulleys or retinacular sheaths. Stenosal tendon sheath results in stimulation by fingers' flexion flequently and inflammatory conditions. Stenosing tenosynovitis is particularly common in diabetic patients. When multiple digits are involved, the possibility of diabetes should be considered in previously undiagnosed patients.

【诊断要点】Keys to diagnosis

(1) 有手部劳损病史，好发于拇指、食指、中指。

Patient has a history of hand strain. Thumb, index and middle fingers are affected commonly.

(2) 拇指、食指和中指活动不灵活，晨起或劳累后症状明显。

Patients feel clumsiness in the thumb, index and middle fingers, in the morning or after overwork.

(3) 掌指关节掌侧压痛，可触及结节，患者手指或拇指伸屈活动困难，有弹响。

Tenderness and nodule are found at palmar aspect of metacarpophalangeal joints. Catching or triggering of the affected finger or thumb is presented by the patient.

【小针刀治疗】Acupotomy therapy

(1) 体位：仰卧位，手掌向上平放于治疗台上（图 2 - 43）。

Posture：Supinate, with palms and wrist on the pillow (Figure 2 - 43).

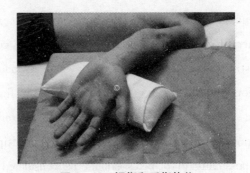

图 2 - 43　拇指和手指体位

Figure 2 - 43　Posture for thumb and finger

（2）定位：拇指及第二至第五指掌指关节掌侧触到硬结处，在该点屈肌腱方向上端、下端各定 1 点，记号笔标记（图 2 - 44）。

Location：An induration being felt in the metacarpophalangeal joint of thumb or in one of finger from the second to the fifth, mark one point in both upper and lower ends of theinduration point along the flexor tendon（Figure 2 - 44）.

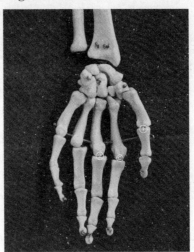

图 2 - 44　屈指肌腱腱鞘炎进针定点

Figure 2 - 44　Inserting points for flexor tenosynovitis

①拇指掌指关节　The metacarpophalangeal joint of thumb；②手指掌指关节 The metacarpophalangeal joint of finger

（3）术野常规消毒，铺巾。

Disinfecting and draping in treatmental area as usual.

（4）针具：Ⅰ型 4 号针刀。

Acupotomy：Type Ⅰ-4 acupotomy.

（5）针刀操作。

Manipulation of acupotomy.

①从硬结的近端进针刀，刀口线与拇长屈肌腱或屈指肌腱走行方向一致，针刀体垂直刺入。通过皮肤、皮下组织，到达腱鞘浅层后再向近端纵向切割，一有落空感即止，范围约 0.5 cm。

An acupotomy is inserted vertically in the proximate of the induration，with the cutting line being in concord with the direction of flexor pollicis longus or flexor digitorum. Through skin and subcutaneous tissue，cutting is performed in the shallow tendon sheath towards the near-end along longitudinal within 0.5 cm range，stopped as soon as felling a falling down.

②从硬结的远端进针刀，刀口线与拇长屈肌腱或屈指肌腱走行方向一致，针刀体垂直刺入。通过皮肤、皮下组织，到达腱鞘浅层后再向远端纵向切割，一有落空感即止，范围约 0.5 cm。

The other acupotomy is inserted vertically in the distal end of the induration，with the cutting line being in concord with the direction of flexor pollicis longus or flexor digitorum. Through skin and subcutaneous tissue，cutting is performed in the shallow tendon sheath towards the far-end along longitudinal within 0.5 cm range，stopped as soon as felling a falling down.

③手术完毕，拨出针刀，局部压迫止血 3 分钟后，用创可贴覆盖针眼。

When acupotomy treatment finished，practitioner withdraws the acupotomy and applies pressure to the treated points for three minutes and adhesive dressing such as a Band-Aid.

注意：进针时，针下有落空感即止，不可切割肌腱硬结，以免损伤肌腱；不可切割或剥离骨面，以免损伤深面的腱系膜，引起术后严重的肿胀和疼痛。

Attention：Stop inserting as soon as felling a falling down to avoid injury of tendons by cutting tendon induration. Do not cut or dissect the bone surface，which may cause damage to mesotendon in the deep layer otherwise it will lead to severe swelling and pain after the treatment.

（6）术后手法。

Manipulation post-acupotomy treatment.

先嘱患者主动屈伸患指数下，然后施术者轻揉牵拉并屈伸其患指数次，切忌使用暴力（图 2 - 45）。

Instruct the patient to bent affected fingers several times，followed by additional times of gentle dragging by the practitioner，beware not to use brute force（Figure 2 - 45）.

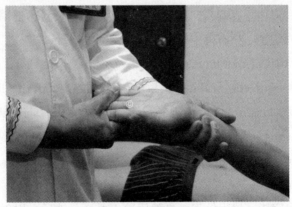

图 2 - 45　指部手法

Figure 2 - 45　Manual manipulation for thumb and finger

16　臀上皮神经卡压综合征　Superior Clunial Nerves Entrapment Syndrome

【概述】 Overview

　　臀上皮神经卡压综合征是臀上皮神经在其越过髂嵴及穿出臀部深筋膜处受牵拉、压迫等损伤而造成的疼痛综合征，主要表现为沿大腿后侧放射至膝关节的持续性疼痛，疼痛部位固定，活动时疼痛加剧。

Superior clunial nerves entrapment syndrome is a pain caused by traction and compression injury of the superior clunial nerves when they passing through crista iliaca and buttock deep fascia. Symptoms include a persistent pain radiating from back side of the thighs to articulation genus and the pain is fixed and increased during activity.

　　臀上皮神经由第一至第三腰椎神经后支之外侧支组成，在股骨大转子与第三腰椎间连线交于髂嵴处平行穿出深筋膜，分布于臀部皮肤，臀上皮神经容易因久弯腰、躯干左右旋转时受到损伤，走行于髂嵴上方的部分神经或纤维束，容易受到磨损，产生水肿充血、神经粗大、无菌性炎症病理状态，造成疼痛。

Consisted of rami lateralis of the 1st to the 3rd rami posteriores nervorum lumbalium, Nervi clunium superiores distribute in hip skin through deep fascia parallel in a connecting line between the greater trochanter of femur and L3 line to the iliac crest. Some of the fibers of those nerves are easily injured at the superior part of the iliac crest by bending or twisting motion of the body, and leading to edema, hyperemia, neural coarsening and inflammation. Painful symptoms are caused by those pathologic facts.

【诊断要点】 Keys to diagnosis

（1）有腰臀部急性闪挫伤或慢性劳损病史。

There is a history of acute sprain or chronic strain in the waist and buttock.

（2）患者常表现为一侧腰臀部疼痛，急性损伤时疼痛较剧，但不会传达至膝部，弯腰活动明显受限。

Patients complain of pain on one side of the waist and buttock. The pain gets severe in acute injury but the pain will be not radiating to the knee. Stooping down movement become obvious limited.

（3）在患者髂前上棘与髂后上棘连线中点及其下方有固定的压痛点，并向同侧大腿后方放射，放射痛不超过膝关节。

Examination finds out fixed tenderness points at patients' midpoint between anterior superior spine and spinal iliaca posterior superior and at the point below. Tenderness may radiate to dorsal part of the thigh but may not radiate down to the knee.

（4）直腿抬高试验多为阴性。

Straight-leg raising test shows negative.

【小针刀治疗】 Acupotomy therapy

（1）体位：俯卧位（图 2 - 46）。

Posture：Prone position (Figure 2 - 46).

（2）定点：髂前上棘与髂后上棘连线中点压痛处（见图 2 - 47）。

Location：Tenderness point in the middle point between anterior superior spine and spina iliaca posterior superior (Figure 2 - 47).

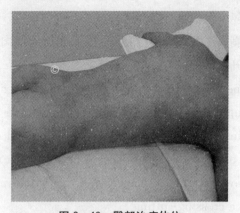

图 2 - 46 臀部治疗体位

Figure 2 - 46 Posture for buttock

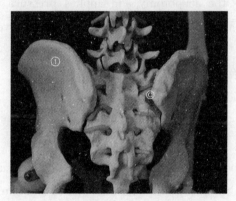

图 2 - 47 臀上皮神经进针定点

Figure 2 - 47 Inserting points for superior clunial nerves

①臀上皮神经进针点 Inserting points for superior clunial nerves

（3）术野常规消毒，铺巾。

Disinfecting and draping in treatmental area as usual.

（4）针具：Ⅰ型 4 号针刀。

Acupotomy：Type Ⅰ-4 acupotomy.

（5）针刀操作。

Manipulation of acupotomy.

刀口线与躯干纵轴平行，针体与进针点皮肤垂直，刺入直达髂骨骨面后先纵行剥离 1 次，再横行剥离 1 次；退针至肌肉筋膜筋结处再行"十"字切开。

Cutting line being in concord with longitudinal axis of the lower limb, and acupotomy body being perpendicular to the skin, an acupotomy is inserted to the surface of the ilium and one seperating broadwise and one dredging lengthwise is performed at the point, and then is withdrawed back to the layer where being spasm of muscle and fascia to make a crossing-cutting.

出针，无菌纱布按压针孔 3～5 分钟，用创可贴覆盖针孔。

Withdraws the acupotomy and applies pressure to the treated points for 3～5 minutes with a sterile gauze and adhesive dressing such as a Band-Aid.

（6）手法治疗。

Manipulation treatment.

针刀术后，患者仰卧位，施术者将其患侧下肢屈髋屈膝活动数次（图 2 - 48）。

After acupotomy treatment: Patient lying on supine position, practitioner makes his/her hip and knee flexed and extend on affected lower limb for several times (Figure 2 - 48).

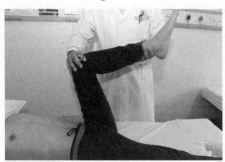

图 2 - 48　臀部手法

Figure 2 - 48　Manual manipulation for buttock

17 梨状肌损伤综合征 Piriformis Injury Syndrome

【概述】Overview

梨状肌损伤综合征是由于梨状肌受到牵拉损伤，引起局部充血、水肿、痉挛，从而刺激或压迫坐骨神经，产生局部疼痛和功能障碍等一系列综合征。

Piriformis injury syndrome is characterized by painful thigh and limited movement caused by piriformis muscle strain leading to stimulation or compression of sciatica resulted from congestion, swollen, spasm in local area.

梨状肌常因髋关节急剧内旋、外旋或外展，感受风寒湿邪等发生损伤、痉挛、肥厚和挛缩，坐骨神经在梨状肌下孔受压引起臀部疼痛和下肢放射痛。

Commonly caused by sharp internal rotation and external rotation, or abduction of hip joint, and the invasion of exogenous pathogenic wind, cold and dampness, piriform muscle is injured and becomes spasm, thicken and cicatrice, which producing painful hip and radiating pain to the leg by compression of nervi ischiadicus at the infrapiriform foramen.

【诊断要点】Keys to diagnosis

（1）自觉臀部一侧酸痛、胀痛，其痛向下沿大腿后方、小腿外后侧放散。严重者，臀部剧痛，下肢伸直困难。

Patient complains of buttocks ached, distended which spread

down to posterior thigh and posterolateral calf. Serious case suffers from pang at buttocks and leg difficult unbending.

（2）咳嗽、打喷嚏或拉大便等增加腹压时，可引起坐骨神经沿走行方向窜痛。

Abdominal pressure increasing such as coughing, sneezing or defecating can produce sciatica.

（3）直腿抬高试验在 60°以前可出现牵拉痛，超过 60°则疼痛反而减轻，此点可与神经根受压作鉴别。

Tractive pain appears when straight leg raising test is less than 60 degrees. The pain would relieve when the test is over 60 degrees, which can differentiate to compression of nerve root.

（4）指压梨状肌部位有明显疼痛，或可能触及紧张的条索状肌束。

Digit pressing at musculi piriformis conduces distinct pain or touch a strip cord like object.

（5）髋关节抗阻力内旋试验呈阳性。

Test of resistance internal rotation of hip joint is positived.

【小针刀治疗】Acupotomy therapy

（1）体位：俯卧位（图 2 - 49）。

Posture：Prone position（Figure 2 - 49）.

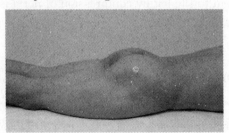

图 2 - 49　臀部治疗体位

Figure 2 - 49　Posture for buttock

（2）定点：梨状肌体表投影的压痛点，即髂后上棘与尾骨尖连线的中点与股骨大转子连线的中内 1/3 交界处（见图 2 - 50）。

Location：Inserting point is the tenderness point which is located in junction between the interior 1/3 and middle 1/3 in projection on body surface of the piriform muscle. This muscle goes from the middle point between the posterior superior iliac spine and the apex of coccyx to the greater trochanter of femur （Figure 2 - 50）.

（3）术野常规消毒，铺巾。

Disinfecting and draping in treatmental area as usual.

（4）针具：Ⅰ型 4 号针刀。

Acupotomy：Type Ⅰ-4 acupotomy.

（5）针刀操作。

Manipulation of acupotomy.

定点处即为进针点，刀口线与坐骨神经走向平行，针刀体与皮肤垂直，刺入后探索进针，当针刀通过臀大肌，达到梨状肌时可能会出现空虚感，调整针尖方向，出现酸胀感处即为病变处，先与梨状肌肌纤维垂直方向切 3 刀，横行剥离 1 次，再纵行疏通 1 次。

As a inserting point mentioned above, blade line being parallel to sciatic nerve, and acupotomy body being perpendicular to the skin, an acupotomy is inserted with searching when it pass through the gluteus maximus, until feeling a falling, indicating the reaching of the piriform muscle. Practitioner tries to find sore point of lesion by adjusting orientation of the needle tip, and performs a three crossing-cutting perpendicular to the muscle fibers of piriform muscle, and then performs one seperating broadwise and one dredging lengthwise at the point.

（6）针刀术后手法治疗。

Manipulation post-acupotomy treatment.

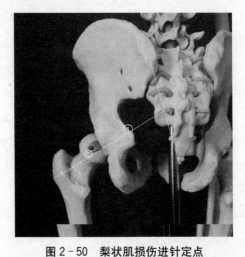

图 2 - 50　梨状肌损伤进针定点

Figure 2 - 50　Inserting points for piriformis injury

①梨状肌进针点　Inserting points for Piriformis

针刀术后，患者仰卧，屈髋屈膝 90°，施术者用手按压住患者膝外侧，嘱患者做外旋抗阻力动作数次（图 2 - 51）。

After acupotomy treatment，patient lying on supine position with hip and knee flexion in 90 degrees，practitioner pushes his/her knee on lateral side while patient extorts his hip to resist for several times (Figure 2 - 51).

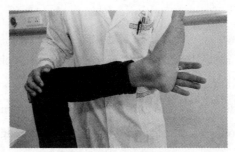

图 2 - 51　臀部手法

Figure 5-51　Manual manipulation for buttock

18　股骨头缺血性坏死　Ischemic Necrosis of the Femoral Head

【概述】Overview

股骨头缺血性坏死是由于股骨头血液循环障碍，引起骨质坏死的病症。

Ischemic necrosis of the femoral head is a disease caused by disturbance of blood circulation of femoral head, which leading to necrosis.

股骨头缺血性坏死病因大致可分为创伤、非创伤和儿童股骨头骨骺缺血性坏死三大类。可由髋关节损伤、关节手术、类风湿性关节炎、饮酒过量、长期激素治疗等多种原因引起。坏死如未能及时修复，可发展为股骨头塌陷，严重影响髋关节功能。

Pathogenic factors of ischemic necrosis of the femoral head can be classified as three kinds including trauma, non-trauma and children ischemic necrosis of capitular epiphysis of femur. It can be caused by hip joint injury, hip joint operation, rheumatoid arthritis, excessive drinking, long-term hormone therapy and other reasons. Femoral head recovery failure promptly leads to developing collapse of the femoral head, and leads to affecting the hip function seriously.

【诊断要点】Keys to diagnosis

（1）患者有髋部外伤史、长期应用激素或酗酒病史。

The patient has a history of hip trauma, long term of taking hormone in a large dose, or excessive drinking.

（2）髋部隐痛，一侧或两侧痛，逐渐加重，跛行、髋关节外展、内外旋活动功能障碍，甚至行走困难。

There is vague pain in one or two hips and the pain get serious gradually. There occur claudication, limitation of abduction, intorsion and extorsion on hip joint. Severe patients have trouble in walking.

（3）患肢缩短，屈髋内收，肌萎缩。"4"字征、托马斯征（Thomas）、艾利斯征（Allis）阳性。

The affected lower extremity became shorter, with flexion, adduction and contracture deformities. There is muscular atrophy. Figure-of-4 test, Thomas' sign and Allis' sign are positive.

（4）影像学检查：FICAT 分类法分为 4 期。

Image examination: There are four stages by FICAT classification.

Ⅰ期：X 射线片无阳性征象，或者只是出现骨质疏松，CT 和 MRI 可见股骨头异常。

Stage Ⅰ: There is no positive sign in X-ray film, or there is osteoporosis only. CT and MRI may show abnormal sign in femoral head.

Ⅱ期：仅侵犯骨骺前部，无塌陷。股骨头边缘有带状硬化带，或者头部有囊状样变，股骨头外形完整。

Stage Ⅱ: Lesion is located at anterior part of the femoral head. There is a hardenability band around edge but is no collapse of femoral head, or there is cystic degeneration in the head but the head form maintain completely.

Ⅲ期：可见边界清晰的骨囊肿状样变，关节间隙有所改变，坏死区密度增高，股骨头边缘出现残缺。

Stage Ⅲ: There are clear bone cyst like changes, joint space change, increase in density of necrotic area and incomplete change around edge of femoral head.

Ⅳ期：侵犯整个骨骺，股骨头塌陷，高度减少，呈扁平状，关节间隙明显变窄或消失。后期 X 射线片可呈骨性关节炎改变。

Stage Ⅳ：Whole epiphysis impingement was found，which showing femoral head collapsed，height decreased，flat shaped and joint space narrowed. X-ray film indicates osteoarthritis changes at the later period.

【小针刀治疗】Acupotomy therapy

（1）体位：前侧入路—仰卧位；外侧入路—侧卧位（图 2 - 52 至图 2 - 54）。

Posture：Anterior approach-supine；lateral approach-lateral position（Figure 2 - 52～Figure 2 - 54）.

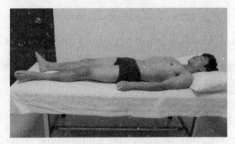

图 2 - 52　髋部前侧入路体位

Figure 2 - 52　Posture for anterior approach of hip

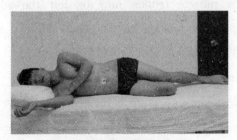

图 2 - 53　髋部外侧入路体位

Figure 2 - 53　Posture for lateral approach of hip

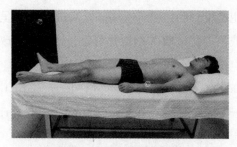

图 2 - 54　髋部治疗体位

Figure 2 - 54　Posture for hip

（2）定点。

Location.

①髋关节前侧关节囊：腹股沟中点下方 2 cm，再向外 2 cm，即股动脉搏动点外侧（图 2 - 55）。

Anterior side of the capsule of hip joint：The point is located 2 cm blow the mid-point of inguinal ligament and then 2 cm lateral, which is lateral of the femoral artery pulsation point（Figure 2 - 55）.

②股内收肌起点：将患者患髋置于屈髋外展位，耻骨结节可触及紧张挛缩的内收肌肌腱处为进针点。

Origin of the adductor muscle：The patient being placed in a position of affected hip flexion and abduction, inserting points are located at the pubic tubercle where muscular tension and contracture of the adductor muscle tendon may be felt the adductor tendon contracture of palpable tension for the needle point.

③外侧：在皮下触及股骨大粗隆最隆起处，向上 3 cm 处定 1 点，两侧旁开 1.5 cm 处各定 1 点，共 3 个点（图 2 - 56）。

Lateral side：The first point is located 3 cm above the top of the femoral intertrochanteric, and two other points are located 1.5 cm on both side of the first point. There are three points totally（Figure 2 - 56）.

116

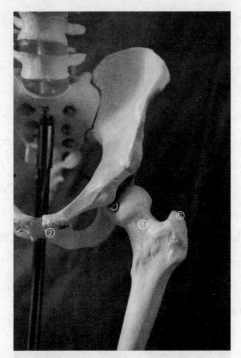

图 2 - 55 髋关节前侧进针定点

Figure 2 - 55 Inserting points for anterior side of the hip joint

①髋关节前侧关节囊 Anterior side of the capsule of hip joint；②股内收肌起点 Origin of the adductor muscle

（3）术野常规消毒，铺巾。

Disinfecting and draping in treatmental area as usual.

（4）针具：Ⅰ型 4 号、Ⅱ型 4 号针刀。

Acupotomy：Type Ⅰ-4 and Ⅱ-4 acupotomy.

（5）针刀操作。

Manipulation of acupotomy.

髋关节前侧关节囊：从髋关节前侧关节穿刺点进针刀，刀口线与下肢纵轴平行，垂直进针，针刀经皮肤、皮下组织，当针刀下有坚韧感时，即到达髂股韧带中部，纵疏横剥 3 刀，范围约 0.5 cm。调转刀

117

口线 90°，向上进针，当有落空感时，即达关节腔，用提插刀法切割 3 刀，范围约 0.5 cm。

Anterior side of the capsule of hip joint: Approaching from anterior side of the capsule of hip joint, cutting line being in concord with longitudinal axis of the lower limb, and acupotomy body being perpendicular to the skin, an acupotomy is inserted through the skin and subcutaneous tissue, until feeling toughed, indicating the reaching of the middle part of iliofemoral ligament. Practitioner first performs a three cut with methods of seperating broadwise and dredging lengthwise, and then turns the blade line 90 degrees and penetrate upwards into articular cavity where falling felling may be felt, and then performs a lifting-thrusting for three times within the range of 0.5 cm.

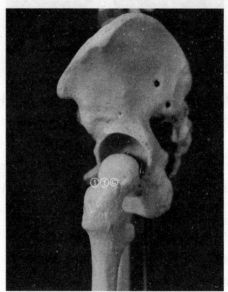

图 2 - 56　髋关节外侧进针定点

Figure 2 - 56　Inserting points for lateral side of the hip joint

①外侧　Lateral side

内收肌起点：从耻骨结节进针刀，刀口线与下肢纵轴平行，垂直进针，针刀经皮肤、皮下组织，向耻骨下支方向行进，刀下有坚韧感时为长收肌起点，切 3 刀，范围 0.5 cm。沿耻骨下支方向向外下行进，刀下有坚韧感时为短收肌、股薄肌起点，贴骨面切 3 刀，范围 0.5 cm。

Origin of the adductor muscle：Inserting from the pubic tubercle，blade line being parallel to and lower longitudinal axis，and acupotomy body being perpendicular to the skin，an acupotomy is inserted through the skin and subcutaneous tissue towards the remi inferior ossis pubis，until feeling toughed，indicating the reaching of the adductor longus. Practitioner first performs a three crossing-cutting，and then turns the needle towards outer lower part of the remi inferior ossis pubis，until feeling toughed，indicating the reaching of the adductor brevis and the gracilis muscle，and then performs a dissecting for three times within the range of 0.5 cm.

外侧：Ⅱ型 4 号针刀，刀口线与下肢纵轴平行，垂直进针，通过皮肤、皮下组织抵达股骨大粗隆，针刀头贴大粗隆上缘刺入，当有落空感时即达关节腔，用提插刀法切割 3 刀，范围 0.5 cm。穿过关节囊，到达股骨颈骨面时，用力将针刀刺入股骨颈骨质中数下。

Lateral side：With a Ⅱ-4 type acupotomy，blade line being parallel to longitudinal axis of lower extremity，and acupotomy body being perpendicular to the skin，practitioner inserts the acupotomy into articular cavity along superior edge of the femoral intertrochanteric where may fell a falling，and performs a three lifting-thrusting within 0.5 cm in length. Performer thrusts the needle deeper through the capsule and surface of bone，and then forces the needle into the bony of femoral neck for several times.

术毕，拔出针刀，局部压迫止血 3 分钟后，用创可贴覆盖针眼。

When acupotomy treatment finished，practitioner withdraws the

119

acupotomy and applies pressure to the treated points for three minutes and adhesive dressing such as a Band-Aid.

（6）针刀术后手法治疗。

Manipulation post-acupotomy treatment.

手法拔伸牵引髋关节后（注意不能旋转关节），在病床上进行间断下肢牵引 6 周，牵引重量为 30 kg，以使关节间隙增宽，血液微循环得以恢复，股骨头有生长空间（图 2 - 57）。

Pull out the affected hip joint by manual traction（without joint rotation），and followed by intermittent traction with 30 kg weight to the affected lower limb for increasing joint space，premoting microcirculation and enlarging a growth space for the femoral head（Figure 2 - 57）.

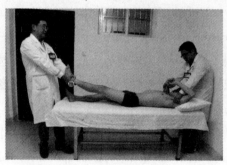

图 2 - 57　髋部手法

Figure 2 - 57　Manual manipulation for hip

19　膝关节侧副韧带损伤　Injury of Collateral Ligament of Knee Joint

【概述】Overview

膝关节外伤致侧方韧带损伤、关节不稳定及疼痛者称为膝关节侧副韧带损伤。

Injuries of collateral ligament of knee joint are caused by trauma on lateral side，leading to instability and pain of the knee joint.

膝关节侧副韧带损伤依据病理变化分为韧带部分撕裂和完全断裂。内侧损伤较外侧常见，若与交叉韧带损伤或半月板损伤同时发生时，则称为膝关节损伤三联症。有的可并发膝关节创伤性滑膜炎。

Injuries of collateral ligament of knee joint are classified to partial tear or complete tear accoding to pathogenic changes. Injuries to the medial ligament are more common than those to the lateral ligaments. These may be associated with cruciate ligaments injuries or meniscal injuries which are called as Triads of knee joint injury. It can be complicated by traumatic synovitis of knee joint in some cases.

【诊断要点】Keys to diagnosis

（1）通常有膝关节外展和扭转受伤史。小腿在外展外翻位受伤，引起膝关节内侧副韧带损伤；在内收内翻位受伤时，则可发生外侧副韧带自腓骨头撕裂。临床以内侧副韧带损伤多见。

A history of abduction injury，often with a torsional component，is usually obtained. Medial collateral ligament injury may wound at position of abduction and ectropion，while knee at position of adduction and ectropion，lateral collateral ligament injury may associated with bony injury of head of fibula. Medial collateral ligament injury is common in clinic.

（2）伤后局部肿胀、疼痛，膝关节不能完全伸直，外展小腿疼痛加剧。合并创伤性滑膜炎者，浮髌试验呈阳性。

After wounded，local part is swelled and painful. Knee joint can not unbend completely. Calf abducts would make pain worse.

121

Floating patella test positive indicates the injury complicated by traumatic synovitis.

（3）如韧带完全断裂，则关节间隙增宽，在韧带损伤处可摸到两断端间的凹陷。

Interspace of joint becomes wider if ligaments are breaked completely. A pitting can be touched at wounded section of ligament between two broken ends.

（4）小腿夹枕 X 射线检查见膝关节间隙增宽（伤侧）。

X-ray film indicates interspace of joint becomes wider （affected side） when the photos are taken in the condition which a pillow is placed between both calfs.

【小针刀治疗】Acupotomy therapy

（1）体位：仰卧位（图 2 - 58）。

Posture：Dorsal position （Figure 2 - 58）.

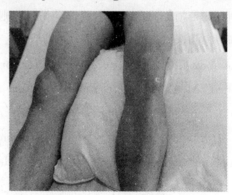

图 2 - 58　膝部治疗体位

Figure 2 - 58　Posture for knee

（2）定点（图 2 - 59）。

Location （Figure 2 - 59）.

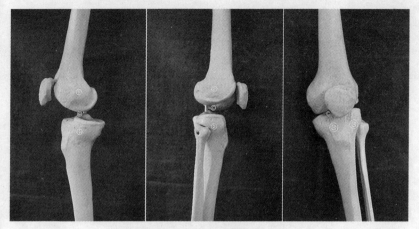

图 2 - 59　膝关节进针定点

Figure 2 - 59　Inserting points for knee joint

①内侧　Medial side；②外侧　Lateral side；③前侧　Anterior side

①内侧：股骨内侧髁胫侧副韧带压痛点、内侧关节间隙压痛点、胫骨上端内侧压痛点。

Medial side：Mark tenderness points at the tibial collateral ligament at the condylus medialis femoris，at medial joint space，and at the medial side of upper end of tibia.

②外侧：股骨外侧髁腓侧副韧带压痛点、外侧关节间隙压痛点、胫骨上端外侧压痛点。

Lateral side：Tenderness points at the fibular collateral ligament at condylus lateralis femoris，at lateral joint space，and at lateral side of upper end of tibia are marked.

③前侧：髌韧带两侧髌下脂肪垫。

Anterior side：Two points are marked for infrapatellar fat pad in both sides of the patellar ligament.

（3）术野常规消毒，铺巾。

Disinfecting and draping in treatmental area as usual.

123

（4）针具：Ⅰ型4号针刀。

Acupotomy：Type Ⅰ-4 acupotomy.

（5）针刀操作。

Manipulation of acupotomy.

内侧：胫侧副韧带的刀口线与下肢纵轴方向一致，针刀体与皮肤垂直，针刀经皮肤、皮下组织，当刀下有韧性感时，即到达内侧副韧带，纵疏横剥3刀。

Medial side：Cutting line at the tibial collateral ligament should be in concord with longitudinal axis of the lower limb, and acupotomy body should be perpendicular to the skin. The acupotomy is inserted through subcutaneous tissue, until feeling toughness, indicating the reaching of medial collateral ligament. Practitioner then performs a three-cut with methods of seperating broadwise and dredging lengthwise at the point.

外侧：腓侧副韧带及髂胫束的粘连和瘢痕，刀口线与下肢纵轴方向一致，针刀体与皮肤垂直，针刀经皮肤、皮下组织，当刀下有韧性感时，即到达腓侧副韧带和髂胫束，纵疏横剥3刀。

Lateral side：Cutting line for adhesion and scar at the fibular collateral ligament and iliotibial band should be in concord with longitudinal axis of the lower limb, and acupotomy body should be perpendicular to the skin. The acupotomy is inserted through subcutaneous tissue, until feeling toughness, indicating the reaching of the fibular collateral ligament and iliotibial band. Practitioner then performs a three-cut with methods of seperating broadwise and dredging lengthwise at the point.

前侧：刀口线与下肢纵轴方向一致，针刀体与皮肤垂直，针刀经皮肤、皮下组织，当刀下有落空感时，即到达髌下脂肪垫，先纵疏横剥3刀，然后斜向对侧脂肪垫方向透刺。

Anterior side: Cutting line being in concord with longitudinal axis of the lower limb, and acupotomy body being perpendicular to the skin, an acupotomy is inserted through subcutaneous tissue, until feeling falling, indicating the reaching of the infrapatellar fat pad. Practitioner first performs a three-cut with methods of seperating broadwise and dredging lengthwise, and then performs a multidirectional penetrating oblique towards the fat pad in opposite side at the point.

（6）术后处理：应早期开始进行股四头肌功能锻炼（图 2 - 60）。

After-treatment: Strengthening the quadriceps should be undertaken in early stage (Figure 2 - 60).

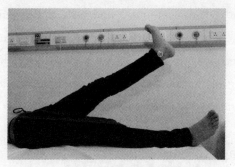

图 2 - 60　股四头肌功能锻炼

Figure 2 - 60　Strengthening the quadriceps

20　膝关节骨性关节炎　Knee Osteoarthritis

【概述】 Overview

膝关节骨性关节炎是一种关节软骨退行性病变，多见于中老年人。临床表现为膝关节疼痛肿胀，活动不灵活，上下楼梯疼痛明显；后期引起膝关节畸形。

Knee osteoarthritis is a chronic articular disorder characterized by degeneration of articular cartilage and is most frequently seen in the middle-aged and old people. Clinical manifestations include pain and swelling in knee joint, limitation of knee motion and pain obviously during walking up and down the stairs. There may be deformity of knee joints in later stage.

中医属"痹证"范畴，主要是由于正气不足，感受风、寒、湿、热之邪而致病。由于膝关节劳损和负重等原因使关节软骨退变和继发性骨质增生，导致关节失稳、关节间隙变窄，引发慢性关节炎症，出现关节疼痛、肿胀、积液、关节活动功能障碍、关节畸形等。

Knee osteoarthritis pertains to the conception of obstructive syndrome in TCM due to insufficiency of vital energe and impingement of pathogenic wind, cold, dampness and heat. Pathogenic factors such as strain and weight bearing of knee result in degeneration of articular cartilage and secondary hyperostogeny leading to instability of the knee joint, narrowing of the joint space, then swelling, joint effusion, joint activity dysfunction and deformity are produced.

【诊断要点】 Keys to diagnosis

（1）膝关节疼痛，行走不便，关节伸屈受限，下蹲及上下楼困难，或突然活动时有刺痛，并常伴有腿软的现象。

Patients complain of painful knee, walking inconvenience, limitation range in knee extension and flexion, difficulty during squatting and walking up and down the stairs, or feel a prick while moving suddenly, and feel a sudden weakness in knee.

（2）膝关节活动受限，并可出现关节积液，浮髌试验呈阳性。

Clinical examination finds out limitation of knee motion and joint effusion. Floating patella test is positive.

（3）X 射线分级标准。

X-ray grading standards.

Ⅰ级：仅有骨刺产生。

Stage Ⅰ：Bony spur can be seen only.

Ⅱ级：关节间隙变窄（少于正常关节间隙的 1/2）。

Stage Ⅱ：Narrowing joint space（1/2 less than the one of normal space）.

Ⅲ级：关节间隙变窄（多于正常关节间隙的 1/2）。

Stage Ⅲ：Narrowing joint space（1/2 more than the one of normal space）.

Ⅳ级：关节间隙消失，或轻度骨磨损（小于 1 cm）。

Stage Ⅳ：Joint space disappear or minor bony worn（less than 1 cm）.

Ⅴ级：重度骨磨损（大于 1 cm），合并半脱位或对侧关节的骨关节炎。

Stage Ⅴ：Severe bony worn（more than 1 cm），associated with subluxation of knee joint or osteoarthritis in the other knee joint.

【小针刀治疗】Acupotomy therapy

（1）体位：仰卧位，膝关节屈曲 30°～45°，膝关节后垫枕（图 2 - 61）。

Posture：Patient is in supine position，with knee joint being bent to 30°～45°，and a bolster behind it（Figure 2 - 61）.

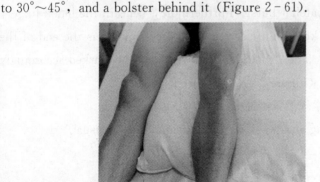

图 2 - 61　膝部治疗体位

Figure 2 - 61　Posture for knee

（2）定位：五指体表定位法。

Location：Five fingers located method.

施术者立于病人体侧，用同侧手做五指定位。如病变在右膝关节，施术者用右手定位；左侧膝关节病变，施术者则用左手定位。掌心正对髌骨中心，五指尽力张开，手指半屈位，中指正对的是髌韧带中部，食指、环指分别对应内膝眼、外膝眼，拇指正对胫侧副韧带起点及股内侧肌下段，小指正对髂胫束行经线上，掌根对准髌上囊。此外，在食指下方，即膝关节间隙下方 4 cm 处向内 3 cm 即为鹅足囊止点。分别用记号笔在上述 7 点定位（图 2 - 62、图 2 - 63）。

The practitioner stands beside the patient，using fingers of the homolateral hand to point. For instance，right side hand should be used for right knee lesion and vice versa. When operating，try to stretch all fingers of the hand to the utmost while center of the palm pointing exactly towards center of the patella；then，the fingers were turned semiflexion，point the middle finger to patellar ligament central，while index finger and ring finger toward inner and outer hsiuen，and the thumb toward start point of the tibial collateral ligament and inferior segment of medial vastus muscle，with little finger pointing meridian line in iliotibial tract，and heel of the hand towards suprapatellar bursa. Furthermore，beneath the index finger，or 4 cm below knee joint clearance and 3 cm inward is the end of the anserine bursa. The 7 mentioned above should be marked accordingly for positioning （Figure 2 - 62、Figure 2 - 63）.

（3）术野常规消毒，铺巾。

Disinfecting and draping in treatmental area as usual.

（4）针具：Ⅰ型 4 号针刀。

Acupotomy：Type Ⅰ-4 acupotomy.

（5）针刀操作。

Manipulation of acupotomy.

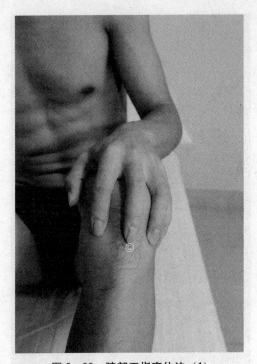

图 2 - 62 膝部五指定位法（1）

Figure 2 - 62 Five fingers located method（1）

胫侧副韧带起点：位于股骨内上髁处，刀口线与下肢纵轴方向一致，针刀体与皮肤垂直，针刀经皮肤、皮下组织，当刀下有韧性感时，即到达胫侧副韧带，先纵疏横剥 3 刀，然后调转刀口线 90°，提插切割 3 刀。

Start point of tibial collateral ligaments：Located in the entepicondyle of femur，cutting line should be in concord with longitudinal axis of the lower limb，and the blade being vertical to skin and subcutaneous tissue，until feeling toughness，indicating the reaching of tibial collateral ligament，the operator should make 3 cuts for dredging lengthwise and seperating broadwise to begin with，then turn the cutting line 90° to cut 3 lines to form "X" with previous cuttings.

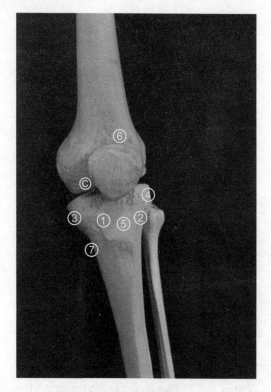

图 2 - 63　膝部五指定位法（2）

Figure 2 - 63　Five fingers located method（2）

①内膝眼　Inner hsiuen；②外膝眼　Outer hsiuen；③胫侧副韧带起点　The tibial collateral ligament；④髂胫束行经线　Meridian linein iliotibial tract；⑤髌韧带　Patellar ligament central；⑥髌上囊　Suprapatellar bursa；⑦鹅足囊止点 The anserine bursa

髌内侧支持带：位于髌骨内侧缘，刀口线与下肢纵轴方向一致，针刀体与皮肤垂直，针刀经皮肤、皮下组织，当刀下有韧性感时，即到达髌内侧支持带，先纵疏横剥 3 刀，然后调转刀口线 90°，"十"字提插切割 3 刀。

Internal patellar ligament：Located in the margin of internal patella, cutting line should be in concord with longitudinal axis of the lower limb, and the blade being vertical to skin and subcutaneous tissue, until feeling toughness, indicating the reaching of internal patellar ligament, the operator should make 3 cuts for dredging lengthwise and seperating broadwise to begin with, then turn the cutting line 90° to cut 3 lines to form "X" with previous cuttings.

髌韧带：位于髌骨尖下方与胫骨粗隆之间，刀口线与下肢纵轴方向一致，针刀体与皮肤垂直，针刀经皮肤、皮下组织，当刀下有韧性感时，即到达髌韧带，进针刀 1 cm，纵疏横剥 3 刀。

Patellar ligament: Located between patella point and tibial tuberositas, cutting line should be in concord with longitudinal axis of the lower limb, and the blade being vertical to skin and subcutaneous tissue, until feeling toughness, indicating the reaching of patellar ligament, then cut a further 1 cm, followed by 3 cuts for dredging lengthwise and seperating broadwise.

髌外侧支持带：位于髌骨外侧缘，刀口线与下肢纵轴方向一致，针刀体与皮肤垂直，针刀经皮肤、皮下组织，当刀下有韧性感时，即到达髌外侧支持带，先纵疏横剥 3 刀，然后调转刀口线 90°，"十"字提插切割 3 刀。

External patellar ligament: Located in the margin of internal patella, cutting line should be in concord with longitudinal axis of the lower limb, and the blade being vertical to skin and subcutaneous tissue, until feeling toughness, indicating the reaching of external patellar ligament, the operator should make 3 cuts for dredging lengthwise and seperating broadwise to begin with, then turn the cutting line 90° to cut 3 lines to form "X" with previous cuttings.

腓侧副韧带及髂胫束：位于股骨外上髁与腓骨头之间，刀口线与下肢纵轴方向一致，针刀体与皮肤垂直，针刀经皮肤、皮下组织，当刀下有韧性感时，即到达腓侧副韧带和髂胫束，纵疏横剥 3 刀。

Fibular collateral ligament and iliotibial tract: Located between external ankle and fibula, cutting line should be in concord with longitudinal axis of the lower limb, and the blade being vertical to skin and subcutaneous tissue, until feeling toughness, indicating the reaching of patellar, then make 3 cuts for dredging lengthwise and seperating broadwise.

股四头肌腱及髌上囊：位于髌骨上缘（髌骨底），刀口线与下肢纵轴方向一致，针刀体与皮肤垂直，针刀经皮肤、皮下组织，当刀下有韧性感时，即到达股四头肌腱，先纵疏横剥 3 刀，再调转刀口线 90°，"十"字提插切割 3 刀，然后继续进针刀，当刀下有落空感时即已穿过股四头肌腱，纵疏横剥 3 刀，范围 0.5 cm。

Tendon of quadriceps femoris and suprapatellar bursa: Located in upper margin (buttom) of the patella, cutting line should be in concord with longitudinal axis of the lower limb, and the blade being vertical to skin and subcutaneous tissue, until feeling toughness, indicating the reaching of the tendon, the operator should make 3 cuts for dredging lengthwise and seperating broadwise to begin with, then turn the cutting line 90° to cut 3 lines to form "X" with previous cuttings; to pass through the tendon, resume inserting until feeling vacant, then repeat dredging lengthwise and seperating broadwise by 3 cuttings within the range of 0.5 cm.

鹅足囊：刀口线与下肢纵轴方向一致，针刀体与皮肤垂直，针刀经皮肤、皮下组织，直达骨面，纵疏横剥 3 刀。

The anserine bursa: Cutting line should be parallel with longitudinal axis of the lower limb, and the blade should be vertical to skin and subcutaneous tissue, practitioner inserts an acupotomy to the bony surface of shin, then performs a three-cut by dredging lengthwise and seperating broadwise by three-cut.

手术完毕，拔出针刀，局部压迫止血 3 分钟后，用创可贴覆盖针眼。

When acupotomy treatment finished，practitioner withdraws the acupotomy and applies pressure to the treated points for 3 minutes and adhesive dressing such as a Band-Aid.

（6）针刀术后手法治疗。

Manipulation post-acupotomy treatment.

患者仰卧，施术者一只手握住踝关节上方，另一只手托住小腿上部，轻柔地伸屈膝关节数次（图 2 - 64）。

Patient lying in supine position，practitioner holds his ankle with one hand and holds his/her shank with the other hand to extend and flex his/her knee joint gentally for several times（Figure 2 - 64）.

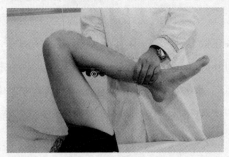

图 2 - 64　膝部手法

Figure 2 - 64　Manual manipulation for knee

21　髌骨软化症　Chondromalacia Patellae

【概述】Overview

髌骨软化症又称髌股关节炎，是由于髌骨软骨面发生软化、关节半脱位，而引起膝部前方疼痛、以上下楼梯时明显的一种常见的膝关节疾病。

Chondromalacia patella is a common disease of knee joint，also called as patellofemoral arthralgia. Because of softening of the patellar cartilage and patellofemoral subluxation, the patients complain of anterior knee pain and the pain becoming obvious during walking up and down the stairs.

髌股关节通常是疼痛的来源，诸如髌骨软骨软化和髌股关节半脱位等，是引起髌股关节痛的主要原因。

The patelolofemoral joint is often the source of pain, entities such as softening of the patellar cartilage and patellofemoral subluxation are main causes of patellofemoral arthralgia.

这类问题的出现是由于髌股关节在半松弛状态时，特别是在关节屈曲0°～20°时。这个范围内关节的失稳源于多种因素，如患者股骨髁的倾角大、存在高位髌骨、退行性变的韧带的过于松弛等。此外，股骨髁前倾度和外翻角度的增大可导致髌股关节不稳定性加大。关节角度的变化将因解剖关系、静态平衡和动态平衡的变化，在髌骨产生接触性高压，压力的增加引发疼痛，并使髌股关节面发生退行性改变。

Many of these problems arise because the patellofemoral joint is semiconstrained, especially in the rage of 0～20 degrees of flexion increases. The degree of constraint is also dependent on a number of othe factors, including the angle of the sulcus of the femur, the presence or absence of patella Alta, and the generalized ligamentous laxity of the patient. In addition, femoral anteversion and increased valgus angle may lead to increased instabiligy of the patellofemoral joint. The degree of congruity may lead to high-contact stresses caused by anatomic configuration and static and dynamic constraints on the patella. Increased pressure may cause pain and degenerative changes in the patellofemoral articular surfaces.

【诊断要点】Keys to diagnosis

（1）有外伤史或劳损病史。

There is a history of being injured or being strained.

（2）髌骨后疼痛，膝软无力，上下楼梯与半蹲位时疼痛加重，可出现"打软腿"或"关节交锁"。

Patient fells painful behind patella and weak in knee. The pain gets worse when going up or down stairs and half-kneeling-squatting. Patient complains "weak knee" or "locked knee".

（3）髌骨研磨试验呈阳性。

Grinding test of patella is positive.

（4）髌下脂肪垫压痛。

Pressure pain is conduced by pressing infrapatellar fat pad.

（5）X射线检查，早期意义不大。晚期可出现髌骨边缘增生或创伤性关节炎改变，或出现关节游离体。

It is meaningless in X-ray examination at early stage. Hyperplasia at edge of patella, or indication of traumatic arthritis, or corpus liberum of joint can be found at radiography.

【小针刀治疗】Acupotomy therapy

（1）体位：仰卧位，膝下垫枕（图 2 - 65）。

Posture：Patient is in supine position，with knee joint being bent to $30°\sim40°$，and a bolster is behind it（Figure 2 - 65）.

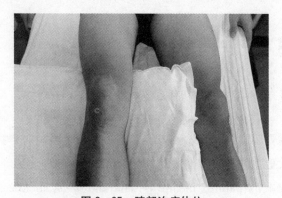

图 2 - 65　膝部治疗体位

Figure 2 - 65　Posture for knee

（2）定点（图 2 - 66）。

Location（Figure 2 - 66）.

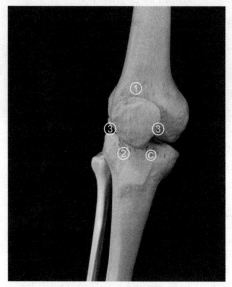

图 2 - 66　髌骨进针定点

Figure 2 - 66　Inserting points for patella

①髌上囊　Suprapatellar bursa；②髌下脂肪垫　The infrapatellar fat pad；
③髌骨内侧、外侧支持带　Retinaculum inside and outside of the patella

①髌上囊：髌骨上缘，即髌骨底上方中点。

Suprapatellar bursa：Superior border of the patella，literally the bottom midpoint beyond the patella.

②髌下脂肪垫：髌骨下缘，即髌骨尖下方髌韧带两侧。

The infrapatellar fat pad：Inferior border of the patella，or patellar ligament in both sides under patella point.

③髌骨内侧、外侧支持带：髌骨内缘、外缘中点。

Retinaculum inside and outside of the patella：Middle point of the interior and superior of the patella.

（3）术野常规消毒，铺巾。

Disinfecting and draping in treatmental area as usual.

（4）针具：Ⅰ型 4 号针刀。

Acupotomy：Type Ⅰ-4 acupotomy.

（5）针刀操作。

Manipulation of acupotomy.

髌上囊：针刀与皮肤垂直，刀口线与下肢纵轴一致，经皮肤、皮下组织，当穿过股四头肌时有落空感，即到达髌上囊，先纵疏横剥 3 刀，然后向后下方膝关节腔透刺 3 刀。

Suprapatellar bursa：The blade being vertical to skin，with the cutting line being in concord with the longitudinal axis of the lower limb，then cut to pass through skin and subcutaneous tissue，until feeling vacant when passing quadriceps femoris. This means the arrival of suprapatellar bursa，and the operator should make 3 cuts for dredging lengthwise and seperating broadwise，followed by 3 thrust cuts in lower part of the knee joint cavity.

髌下脂肪垫：刀口线与下肢纵轴方向一致，针刀体与皮肤垂直，针刀经皮肤、皮下组织，当刀下有落空感时，即到达髌下脂肪垫，先纵疏横剥 3 刀，然后斜向对侧脂肪垫方向透刺 3 刀。

The infrapatellar fat pad: Cutting line being in concord with the longitudinal axis of the lower limb, and the blade being vertical to skin and subcutaneous tissue, until feeling vacant when reaching, then the operator should make 3 cuts for dredging lengthwise and seperating broadwise, followed by 3 thrust cuts oblique to Fat pad underneath the patella.

髌骨内侧、外侧支持带：刀口线与下肢纵轴方向一致，针刀体与皮肤垂直，针刀经皮肤、皮下组织，当刀下有韧性感时，即到达髌内（外）侧支持带，先纵疏横剥3刀，然后调转刀口线90°，"十"字提插切割3刀。

Retinaculum inside and outside of the patella: Cutting line being in concord with the longitudinal axis of the lower limb, and the blade being vertical to skin and subcutaneous tissue, until reaching the retinaculum inside/outside of the patella, the operator should make 3 cuts for dredging lengthwise and seperating broadwise to begin with, then turn the cutting line 90° to cut 3 lines to form "X" with previous cuttings.

（6）针刀术后手法治疗。

Manipulation post-acupotomy treatment.

施术者轻柔的屈伸患者患侧膝关节数次，并在其膝关节伸直位用双手拇指将髌骨向膝关节内侧推压（图2-67）。

Practitioner performs flexion and extension gently in patient's affected knee joint, and then pushes his/her patella inward with both thumbs while patient's knee in extended position (Figure 2-67).

注意：由于髌骨软骨软化，不宜进行髌骨直接按摩，以免加重关节面摩擦损伤。

Attention: Because chondromalacia patellae, massage at patella directly should be avoided in order not to increase damage of facies articularis.

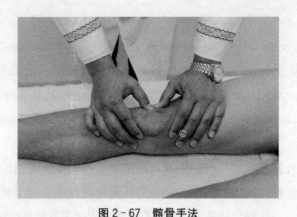

图 2 - 67 髌骨手法

Figure 2 - 67 Manual manipulation for patella

（7）术后处理。

After-treatment.

患者应避免半蹲位与负重，坚持直腿抬高锻炼，开展股四头肌舒缩锻炼，防止肌肉萎缩。

Patient ought to avoid half-kneeling-squatting and weight bearing and should keep exercise of straight-leg raising, contract musculi quadriceps femoris to prevent muscles atrophy.

22 踝关节陈旧性损伤 Obsolete Injury of Ankle Joint

【概述】Overview

本病是指踝关节陈旧性韧带扭伤或撕裂而出现踝部疼痛，活动不便。可发生于任何年龄，尤以运动员发病较多，如果是韧带撕裂，则可有内翻畸形、外翻畸形。临床上以足内翻致外踝韧带损伤较为常见。

Obsolete injuries of ankle joint refer to ankle pain and

inconvenient activity result in chronic ankle ligaments sprain or ligaments tear. These injuries may happen in any ages and are most frequently seen in the athlete. Enstrophe or ectropion deformity of ankle joint can be found if there is ligament tear. It is more common that lateral collateral ligament injury in ankle enstrophe position in the clinic.

由于外侧副韧带扭伤的频发，踝关节周围其他重要结构的损伤常被误诊为一般的踝关节扭伤。踝关节韧带可与外侧副韧带联合损伤或单独损伤。三角联合韧带损伤也容易因注意力过于集中于外侧副韧带而被忽略，三角韧带扭伤的失治可成为踝关节功能障碍久治不愈的原因。

Because of the frequency of lateral collateral ligament sprains，injuries to other important structures around the ankle are often misdiagnosed as routine ankle sprains. Ligaments of ankle joint may be injured in conjunction with lateral collateral sprains or as isolated injuries. Deltoid ligament complex injuries may also be overlooked as attention is focused on the lateral ligaments. A deltoid sprain can be a source of long-term disability if left untreated.

急性损伤后引起踝关节周围软组织出血、水肿，最终形成粘连瘢痕、韧带挛缩，严重者引起踝关节强直。

After acute injury of ankle，soft tissues around ankle joint become hemorrhage，edema leading to lesions such as adhesion，cicatrice and contracture of ligaments at last. Arthrocleisis of ankle joint can be seen in severe case.

【诊断要点】 Keys to diagnosis

（1）有明确的踝内翻或外翻扭伤史。

There is a obvious sprain history on ankle enstrophe or ankle ecstrophy.

（2）踝关节内外侧疼痛、肿胀、压痛、跛行。足内翻时，引起外侧韧带部位疼痛；足外翻时，引起内侧韧带部位疼痛。

Pain, swelling, tenderness and limp can be presented in ankle joint. Pain may appear in lateral collateral ligament when the ankle being enstrophe; while pain may appear in medial collateral ligament when the ankle being ecstrophy.

（3）X 射线检查排除骨折和脱位。

X-ray can exclude any fracture and dislocation.

【小针刀治疗】Acupotomy therapy

（1）体位：仰卧位（图 2 - 68）。

Posture: Dorsal position (Figure 2 - 68).

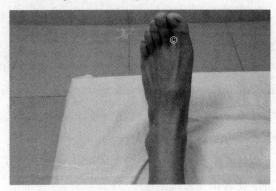

图 2 - 68　踝部治疗体位

Figure 2 - 68　Posture for ankle

（2）定点（图 2 - 69）。

Location (Figure 2 - 69).

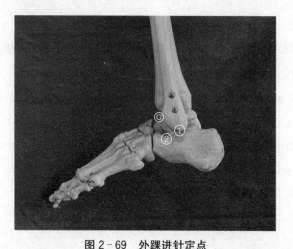

图 2 - 69　外踝进针定点

Figure 2 - 69　Inserting points for external malleolus

①外踝尖三角韧带　Ligamenta deltoideum at tip of the outer ankle bone；

②伸肌下支持带　Inferior extensor retinaculum

①外踝：外踝尖三角韧带及其远端 1 cm 的伸肌下支持带外侧下部各定 1 点。

External malleolus：One point is marked at insertion of ligamenta deltoideum at the tip of the outer ankle bone；the other point is marked at 1 cm below the outer ankle bone where the inferior extensor retinaculum located.

②内踝：内踝尖上 2 cm 处伸肌下支持带上束和内踝尖下 2 cm 处伸肌下支持带下束各定 1 点（图 2 - 70）。

Medial malleolus：One point is marked at upper branch of inferior extensor retinaculum；the other point is marked at 2 cm below the medial malleolus where lower branch of the inferior extensor retinaculum located（Figure 2 - 70）.

③前侧：踝关节平面、足背动脉外侧 1 cm 处，趾长伸肌腱鞘定第 1 点。

Anterior side: On the level of ankle joint, the first point is chosen at tendinous sheath of extensor digitorum longus which located 1 cm lateral to the dorsalis pedis.

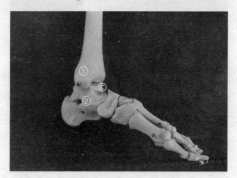

图 2 - 70 内踝进针定点

Figure 2 - 70 Inserting points for medial malleolus

①内踝尖伸肌下支持带上束 Upper branch of inferior extensor retinaculum;

②内踝尖伸肌下支持带下束 Lower branch of the inferior extensor retinaculum

④踝关节平面、足背动脉内侧 1 cm 处，拇长伸肌腱鞘上部定第 2 点。

The second point is marked at 1 cm interior to the dorsalis pedis where the upper part of vagina tendinis musculi extensoris pollicis longi located in level of ankle joint.

在第 2 点远端 2 cm，足背动脉内侧 1 cm 处，拇长伸肌腱鞘下部定第 3 点（见图 2 - 71）。

The third point for lower part of vagina tendinis musculi extensoris pollicis longi is marked 2 cm to the distal end from the second point and 1 cm inferior to the dorsalis pedis (Figure 2 - 71).

（3）术野常规消毒，铺巾。

Disinfecting and draping in treatmental area as usual.

（4）针具：Ⅰ型 4 号针刀。

Acupotomy: Type Ⅰ-4 acupotomy.

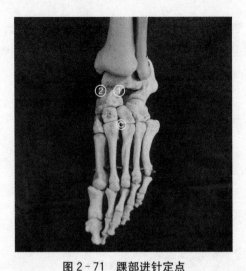

图 2-71　踝部进针定点

Figure 2-71　Inserting points for ankle

①前侧：踝关节平面、足背动脉外侧 1 cm 处，趾长伸肌腱鞘　Anterior side：On the level of ankle joint，tendinous sheath of extensor digitorum longus which located 1 cm lateral to the dorsalis pedis；②踝关节平面、足背动脉内侧 1 cm处，拇长伸肌腱鞘上部　Level of ankle joint：1 cm interior to the dorsalis pedis where the upper part of vagina tendinis musculi extensoris pollicis longi located

（5）针刀操作。

Manipulation of acupotomy.

外踝：刀口线与小腿纵轴方向一致，针刀体与皮肤呈 90°，从外踝定点处刺入，针刀经皮肤、皮下组织，当刀下有阻力感，即到达伸肌下支持带上部的粘连瘢痕，提插刀法切割 3 刀，深度达骨面，然后纵疏横剥 3 刀，范围约 0.5 cm。

External malleolus：With the edge line direction of the acupotomy being parallel to the shank axis and the body of the acupotomy being perpendicular to the skin, a practitioner inserts an acupotomy at the selected point in external malleolus, through the skin, subcutaneous tissue, and fascia to the bone surface of adhesion and cicatrice in inferior extensor retinaculum, where sense of resistance can be felt at the acupotomy tip, he then performs a three-cut with methods of seperating broadwise and dredging lengthwise within 0. 5 cm in length.

内踝：刀口线与小腿纵轴方向一致，针刀体与皮肤呈 90°，从内踝定点处刺入，针刀经皮肤、皮下组织，当刀下有阻力感时，即到达伸肌下支持带上部的粘连瘢痕，提插刀法切割 3 刀，深度达骨面，然后纵疏横剥 3 刀，范围约 0.5 cm。

Malleolus medialis: With the edge line direction of the acupotomy being parallel to the shank axis and the body of the acupotomy being perpendicular to the skin, a practitioner inserts an acupotomy at the selected point in malleolus medialis, through the skin, subcutaneous tissue, and fascia to the bone surface of adhesion and cicatrice in inferior extensor retinaculum, where sense of resistance can be feeled at the acupotomy tip, he then performs a three-cut with methods of seperating broadwise and dredging lengthwise within 0. 5 cm in length.

前侧：刀口线与伸肌腱方向一致，针刀体与皮肤呈 90°，从定点刺入，针刀经皮肤、皮下组织，当刀下有阻力感时，即到达趾长伸肌腱鞘或拇长伸肌腱腱鞘的粘连瘢痕，继续进针刀 1 cm，纵疏横剥 3 刀，范围约 0.5 cm。

Anterior side: With the edge line direction of the acupotomy being parallel to extensor tendon and the body of the acupotomy being perpendicular to the skin, a practitioner inserts an acupotomy at the selected point, through the skin and subcutaneous tissue to lesion of adhesion and cicatrice in the vaginae tendinum musculi extensoris digitorum pedis longi or the extensor pollicis longus tendon sheath, where sense of resistance can be felt at the acupotomy tip, he then inserts the needle 1 cm deeper to performs a three-cut with methods of seperating broadwise and dredging lengthwise within 0.5 cm in length.

术毕，拔出针刀，局部压迫止血 3 分钟后，用创可贴覆盖针眼。

When acupotomy treatment finished, practitioner withdraws the acupotomy and applies pressure to the treated points for three minutes and adhesive dressing such as a Band-Aid.

（6）针刀术后手法治疗。

Manipulation post-acupotomy treatment.

在助手的协助下行踝关节的对抗性牵引，使关节充分背屈、跖屈数次后，施关节弹压术以促使关节恢复到正常角度（图 2 - 72）。

With the help of an assistant doing confrontational traction in patient's ankle joint, practitioner makes patient's ankle full extended and flexed for several times, and then pushes the ankle with a spring force to replace that ankle joint to normal angle (Figure 2 - 72).

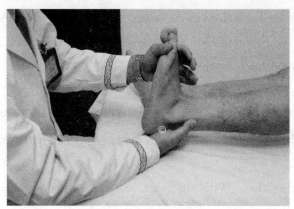

图 2 - 72　踝部手法

Figure 2 - 72　Manual manipulation for ankle

23　跟痛症　Heel Pain（Calcaneodynia）

【概述】 Overview

跟痛症常发于跟部蹠面及跟部后侧，以足跟痛、走路时加重为主诉，与跟骨周围组织慢性劳损和退行性变有关，多发生于老年肥胖之人。

Heel pain（Calcaneodynia）usually occurs on the plantar aspect of the heel but may also occur on the posterior aspect. Complaints include pain on heel and the pain getting worse during walk due to chronic strain and degeneration of the tissue around calcaneus. It mostly occurs in fat and old people.

当评估患者足跟痛时，临床医生必须尽可能准确地判断病位和疼痛的原因。由于病因相当多样性，需要仔细判定，以便选择合适的治疗方案。

When evaluating the patient for heel pain, the clinician must attempt to define as precisely as possible the location and，hence，the cause of the pain.

足跟蹠底部疼痛的病因有蹠腱膜炎、足跟垫萎缩、创伤后因素（如跟骨骨折）、跟骨骨刺的增大、神经因素如跗管综合征、椎间盘退变疾病至足跟的放射痛、系统性疾病（如瑞特氏综合征、银屑病关节炎）、急性蹠腱膜损伤、跟骨结节炎等。然而，跟骨后侧痛的病因包括跟骨后滑囊炎和跟腱止点退行性变等。

Causes of plantar heel pain include plantar fasciitis，atrophy of heel pad，posttraumatic（e. g.，calcaneal fracture），enlarged calcaneal spur，neurologic conditions such as tarsal tunnel syndrome，degenerative disk disease with radiation toward heel, systemic disease (e. g. , Reiter's syndrome, psoriatic arthritis), acute tear of plantar facia, calcaneal apophysitis. However, the causes of posterior heel pain include retrocalcaneal bursitis and degeneration of Achilles tendon insertion.

【诊断要点】Keys to diagnosis

(1) 无明显原因出现足跟痛，尤以早晨起床后站立时痛显，稍活动后减轻。

Painful heel takes place unreasonable. The pain is obvious when getting up and touching ground in the morning, but gets relieved after walking a while.

(2) 足跟痛局部无肿胀，但压痛明显。

There is not any swelling at spot of painful heel, but there is distinct pressure pain.

(3) 行高低不平地面时患足跟疼痛加剧。

Affected heel gets much painful when walking on concavo-convex ground.

(4) X 射线片部分提示跟骨骨刺形成。

X-ray film indicates spur at heel bone in some cases.

【小针刀治疗】Acupotomy therapy

(1) 体位：俯卧位（图 2 - 73）。

Posture：Prone position (Figure 2 - 73).

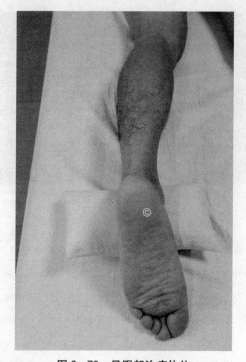

图 2 - 73　足跟部治疗体位

Figure 2 - 73　Posture for heel

（2）定点（图 2 - 74）。

Location（Figure 2 - 74）.

①跟骨结节前缘与足底外侧 1/3 交界处，跖腱膜止点处压痛点。

At the junction of the anterior side of the tuberosity of the calcaneus and one third of the lateral side of the sole，the tenderness point at the ending of the plantar aponeurosis.

②跟骨结节内缘压痛点。

Tenderness at the interior edge of plantar fascia should be chosen，too.

（3）术野常规消毒，铺巾。

Disinfecting and draping in treatmental area as usual.

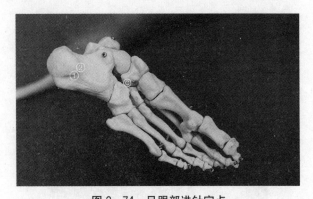

图 2 - 74　足跟部进针定点

Figure 2 - 74　Inserting points for heel

①跟骨结节前缘与足底外侧 1/3 交界处，跖腱膜止点处压痛点　At the junction of the anterior side of the tuberosity of the calcaneus and one third of the lateral side of the sole，the tenderness point at the ending of the plantar aponeurosis；②跟骨结节内缘压痛点　Tenderness at the interior edge of plantar fascia

（4）针具：Ⅰ型 4 号针刀。

Acupotomy：Type Ⅰ-4 acupotomy.

（5）针刀操作。

Manipulation of acupotomy.

跟骨结节前缘：从跟骨结节前缘与足底外侧 1/3 交界处压痛点进针，刀口线与跖腱膜方向一致，针刀体与皮肤呈 90°，针刀经皮肤、皮下组织、脂肪垫，到达跟骨结节前缘骨面，调转刀口线 90°，在骨面上向前下切 3 刀，范围 0.5 cm。

Anterior edge of tuber calcanei: With the edge line direction of the acupotomy being parallel to the plantar fascia and the body of the acupotomy being perpendicular to the skin，a practitioner inserts an acupotomy at the bone surface of the anterior edge of tuber calcanei，he then turns the acupotomy 90 degrees to perform 3 cuttings along

150

the bone surface within 0. 5 cm in length.

跟骨结节内缘：针刀从跟骨结节内缘的压痛点进针，刀口线与跖腱膜方向一致，针刀体与皮肤呈 90°，针刀经皮肤、皮下组织、脂肪垫，到达跟骨结节内缘骨面，调转刀口线 90°，在骨面上向前下切 3 刀，范围约 0. 5 cm，以松解跖腱膜的内侧部。

Interior edge of tuber calcanei: With the edge line direction of the acupotomy being parallel to the plantar fascia and the body of the acupotomy being perpendicular to the skin, a practitioner inserts an acupotomy at the bone surface of the interior edge of tuber calcanei, he then turns the acupotomy 90 degrees to perform 3 cuttings along the bone surface within 0. 5 cm in length for releasing interior side of the plantar fascia.

术毕，拔出针刀，局部压迫止血 3 分钟后，用创可贴覆盖针眼。

When acupotomy treatment finished, practitioner withdraws the acupotomy and presses the points for 3 minutes to stop bleeding, covers points with Band-Aid.

注意：针刀治疗跟痛症是对挛缩的跖腱膜进行松解，不是用针刀去刮除、切断骨刺。

Attention: Aim of acupotomy treatment for heel pain is to release contracture of the plantar fascia instead of striking off or cutting off the bony spur.

（6）针刀术后手法治疗。

Manipulation post-acupotomy treatment.

针刀术毕，嘱患者俯卧位，施术者双手握足底前部，嘱患者踝关节尽量背伸，在背伸到最大位置时，术者用力将踝关节背伸 1 次（图 2 - 75）。

After the acupotomy treatment, patient lying in pronate position and extending his ankle as he can, practitioner holds patient's anterior part of foot with both hands and gives a push to the pelma with force when the patient making his/her ankle to its fullest extent（Figure 2 - 75）.

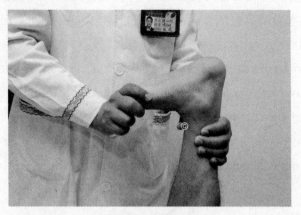

图 2 - 75　跟部手法

Figure 2 - 75　Manual manipulation for heel